FAT-ME NOT

Weight Loss Diet of The Future

Myo M Nwe, MD
Sandeep Grewal, MD

Ace Innovation Group
Aye T Myo, MS
744 Arden Lane, Suite 100
Rock Hill, SC 29732
803-325-2236 ext 237

www.fat-me-not.com

Ordering Information:

Special discounts are available on quantity purchases by corporations, associations, and others. For details, contact the publisher at the address above.

Orders by U.S. trade bookstores and wholesalers please contact to Aye Myo @ 803-325-2236 Ext 237

Printed in the United States of America

Publisher's Cataloging-in-Publication data

Authors: Myo M Nwe, MD
Sandeep Grewal, MD
Title: Fat-Me-Not: Weight Loss Diet of the Future

Illustrator: James-illus
Book design: Jana, impact studios

ISBN: 978-0-9909247-0-8 (Hard Cover)
ISBN: 978-0-9909247-1-5 (Paperback Black/ white)
ISBN: 978-0-9909247-2-2 (Paperback Full Color)
ISBN: 978-0-9909247-3-9 (Digital)

First Edition 2014

Follow us on twitter :

>https://twitter.com/SlimPlate

Like us on facebook :

>https://www.facebook.com/SlimPlate

Read weight loss blog by Dr Nwe at :

>www.aceweightloss.com

Register Dr. Nwe's Online Weight Loss Program at :

>http://www.slimplatesystem.com/register

PREFACE

There is a lot of research being done on weight loss in scientific labs all over the world, but there is still a big disconnect between what scientists are finding out about weight-loss and what consumers are being told. Why is this? Scientists are more inclined to write research papers than to simplify their research for regular consumers who could benefit from the research. Also those who are educating people about weight loss, or making products for it, are not in touch with the latest research on weight loss. The result is that weight loss advice and products on the market in 2014 reflect the scientific advances of 1960s, completely ignoring the giant strides made more recently in this field by scientists who have toiled in the lab and by lab rats whose stories will open a new window into the amazing world of weight loss and how to do it right.

We wrote this book to update your knowledge on the latest scientific evidence and research on weight loss and clarify how our body maintains weight and how you can lose weight. The book also debunks several myths about weight loss, which until now have been the pillars of the weight loss industry.

Either you are trapped in a FAT-ME-YES cycle and are unable to lose weight no matter what you do, or, if you're lucky, you are in the FAT-ME-NOT cycle of life and are able to stay slim and maintain your weight. But the chances are that you really don't know how or why this is happening. The information in this book will blow your mind away and shake the very foundation of your weight loss concept.

But before we start, let's honor those lab rats that have sacrificed their health, happiness, and even their lives to give us a deeper understanding about obesity, weight gain and loss, and how we can be healthy.

Enjoy!

Myo M. Nwe, MD
Sandeep S Grewal, MD

Table of Contents

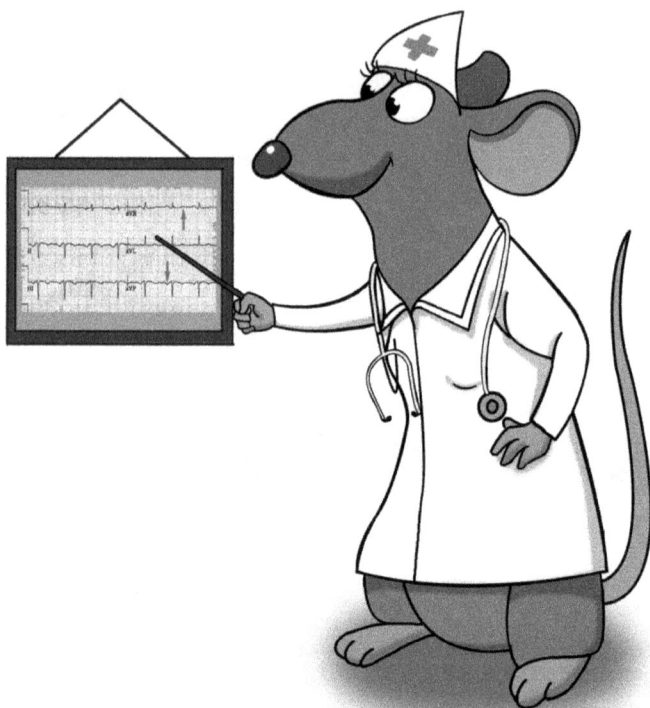

"Fat-Me-Not"

Chapter 1
Why I Wrote This Book?

Being a doctor

I am a practicing Primary Care Physician at Ace Medical Group in Rock Hill, South Carolina. I have practiced medicine since 2003 and obesity medicine since 2007.

Having a patient-doctor relationship is the part of my profession; I take the most pride in. The patient-doctor relationship is different from any other relationships; it is different from relationships with family, friends, or colleagues.

There is an immediate, invisible, but whole heart-felt **bond** between doctor and patient. It's rare that people so immediately reveal things about themselves to any other person than a doctor. But between a doctor and a patient, the patient will tell the doctor their innermost fears instantly.

"Doctor, I cannot breathe," one patient told me. "It started when I had a car accident on I-77. I fear that these dividers are too close to me and too tight. I cannot breathe. I want to pull up and run out of the car."

People feel comfortable telling their inner secrets to a doctor. As a doctor, I know how doctors feel, too. They treat their patients' conditions with kindness and respect. This is a mutual, instantly formed, lovely bond.

There is a strong **trust** between a patient and the doctor. The patient entrusts the doctor with their most secretive matters — even their lives.

"I've had this patch of rash for two weeks," another patient said to me. "I might have done something wrong. I went out with this stranger, I didn't use protection, and..."

As a doctor, anything a patient tells me goes into my inner-most memory, where I lock it in. Doctors are trained not to talk about private matters with any third party and protect their patients' secrets.

Then there is **obedience** from the patient, wherein the doctor's advice is usually taken into the patients' heart.

It is a proven fact that people tend to quit smoking cigarettes and go on weight loss plans when their doctors ask them to do so. People are more likely to listen to their doctor.

And you know what? The same thing applies to doctors, too. As a doctor, I might be able to ignore anyone else's phone call, but my patients' calls must be answered. I know that I must wake up in the middle of the night sometimes to answer that phone call.

I stay very busy in the daytime, so the moment I get in the car to go home, I go over my mental checklist to see if I've forgotten to attend to any patient's need. The patient-doctor relationship doesn't stop at the end of the business day, nor should it.

Hope light up in a patient's eyes, even when hope is only a dim light at the end of the tunnel.

Every time, we fight cancer or any terminal illness, hope shines from the patient's eyes. They don't have longing for hope from other family members, friends or relatives, only from their doctor. The few minutes they have with their doctor, when the doctor comes in and talks to them, make the patients' day. They're eager to hold on to the hope and they trust their doctor will help them keep that hope alive.

At the same time, doctors are conscious of this heroic moment in which they are responsible for deciding what to do and say that will be best for their patients. As doctors, we want to pull all the strings to get mountains to move and keep hope alive. This feeling is always there. I may not always experience this need to play the hero for my patients, but there are times when I feel incredibly responsible for providing my patients with a relief or a cure.

And, finally, there is long-lasting **love**. There is no need for a promise to keep or the need to reiterate this feeling; we know regardless.

I don't play the lottery; I never even imagine myself so rich that I don't need to work. There's a reason for this. I don't need money. Even if I were a multi-millionaire, I'd still be called to practice medicine, working with patients and touching their lives every single day.

What my day looks like

As I mentioned earlier, every day I see 20 plus patients in the clinic as well as 4-8 patients in the nearby hospital. With the exception of vacations, this has been the case every day of the year since I first joined Ace Medical Group as a doctor in 2006.

It's important to me to see my patients not only when they are well, but also when they are so sick that they have to go to the hospital.

So you can see how much I enjoy what I do.

My childhood

I was a curious, well-read kid; as a teenager I won awards and worked incredibly hard; and I was a goal-achieving college student. I acquired my medical degree from a very prestigious school called the Institute of Medicine in Rangoon, Burma. Entrance into the school was extremely competitive, and at that time the three medical schools in Burma only produced 500 physicians annually.

I grew up in a loving family and I am very loving towards my family and friends.

My career

After graduation, I came to the United States. I then continued with my career here; I passed the required exams and completed my residency in New York City before moving down to Rock Hill, South Carolina in 2003.

My interest in Obesity

During my internship, my interest in obesity was piqued. When we discharged a patient from the hospital, we had to hand-write all prescriptions, one medication per script. I had to write the patient's name, age, date of birth, and address as well as my name, the name of my attending, my license number, etc., for every single prescription.

If you don't already know, the internship is one of the busiest times in a doctor's life; you can only imagine how much of a toll it took on me. Every single time I prepared prescriptions, I thought about how to combine all these medications into one medication.

Even though I was unable to create a single magic pill to treat all diseases like high blood pressure, diabetes, high cholesterol, arthritis, and sleep apnea, I noticed a common fact that many of the patients who take multiple medications also carry unhealthy weight. The more I observed, the more I realized that excessive pounds on them were demanding these medications. These patients became frequent fliers to the hospitals. I used to play a little prediction game. I'd look at the weight of a person and I'd guess the number of medications they took.

You got it right! They go hand-in-hand. The greater the weight, the greater the number of medications.

Practicing medicine and practicing weight-loss medicine

After my residency in 2003, I initially joined a larger group practice for few years. Then, in 2006, I co-founded the Ace Medical Group. Three months later, I co-founded the Ace Medical Weight Loss Center.

Here, I want to share the weight loss journey of my patients and myself. We have been through many phases of weight loss treatment we offered through our weight loss center, including multiple meal replacements and different diet plans like low carb, low fat, and low calories. We met many challenges along the way, and success was a long time coming.

In late 2008, we scratched all of our treatment protocols. We started the portion control technique for weight loss based on the most popular and successful techniques for long-term weight loss in our weight-loss center. I drew out multiple portion control plates and tools. We started a group weight loss boot camp, where we did group counseling using the portion plates. We created a sandwich belt, and different belts for different food items. We separated different calories for men and women and used different levels on the bowls for different items as well as different levels on the drinks.

In 2009, we perfected this systematic portion control weight-loss system. It's called the SlimPlate System. The product from start to finish is very different, as the final product now is very easy and intuitive.

Soon after the initial marketing of the SlimPlate System we needed to order a second, larger container due to the demand. That's when we reevaluated the System. It was thoroughly considered from different angles, including science, user friendliness and sustainability; however, we didn't find anything else to improve aside from the addition of a portion spoon and fork.

In February 2013, we successfully launched the SlimPlate System online at www.slimplatesystem.com.

In January 2014, we launched the SlimPlate Online Weight-Loss Program and offered it free, which takes place over the course of four months, an at-home weight-loss program. The program takes our customers through the step-by-step practical approach of a successful weight-loss journey. You can enroll in the program for free at http://www.slimplatesystem.com for a limited time.

In 2014, I completed this book "Fat-Me-Not" to guide patients through the right way of losing weight and keeping it off.

When I was younger, my father said about me "If she wants something, she will not even breathe that the breathing might delay it."

My husband always says, "She always has to get what she wants."

I am very persistent.

Here is my mission: "We've got to win this obesity battle."

My eyes are on it.

My heart is in it.

My thoughts are on it.

I often dream about it.

I sleep on it.

The name of this book came to me in my sleep.

So my question is: "Are you with me?"

Losing weight is not hard, but it is important to start right. Otherwise you will get lost in the cycle of weight gain and weight loss.

Here, therefore, is "Fat-Me-Not": The Weight Loss Diet of the Future.

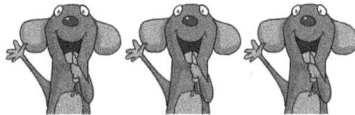

Chapter 2

Weight Loss is Not Logical, It is Biological

Busting The 10 Myths of Weight Loss.

Myth #1:   **If you do not eat, you will lose weight**

Myth #2:   **If you only eat once a day, you will lose weight**

Myth #3:   **Diet sugar and diet drinks are good for losing weight**

Myth #4:   **Fast food is bad, but fine dining is okay**

Myth #5:   **Eating salad and grilled chicken is the way to go
            for weight loss**

Myth #6:   **Exercise is everything to weight loss**

Myth #7:   **Eating carbs will make you fat**

Myth #8:   **Switch from caffeinated to decaffeinated to lose weight**

Myth #9:   **Eating sweets, desserts, and chocolate are no-noes
            for weight loss**

Myth #10: **Obesity is healthy and there is nothing wrong with it**

Weight loss is biological. It defies logic and is not logical. Why? Because we still do not have complete understanding of how our body uses food. Here are some logical sounding diets.

- Jaw wiring diet
- Tongue patch diet
- Fat melt-away cream
- Weight-loss shake powder
- Weight-loss sprayer
- Take one magic pill for weight loss
- Fat blocker
- Detoxes and cleansing
- Skipping meals one day completely
- Eating only meat one day per week

Our patients share many interesting things with us in the group session.

"I was advised that if my weight loss stalled, that I should eat only protein for one day out of the week."

"I was advised to only eat half of the plate."

"I was advised to eat only vegetables — to become a vegetarian."

Though it's easy to look at the above and think of it as logical, the truth is that it's wrong: it's not biological.

It sounds reasonable that we only taste food in a two-inch area of our tongues. Why not cover it up and surely we won't eat as much!

It sounds right that eating is only possible by opening the mouth. So let's wire the jaw so food can't get in!

It sounds reasonable that since we can feel the extra fat right on the surface; a magical rub surely will make that fat just melt away.

If it sounds like there's one trick and only one thing to do, then it's not right for weight loss. Weight loss isn't about "not eating," and choosing not to eat isn't the right way to go about losing weight either.

These techniques all sound logical because we're all eager to get our lean body now — not in three months, but now.

I completely understand: I want it now, too.

But let's think about this for a moment. Is it true? Is it biological? Is this how our body works?

Is it biological?

There are three germ layers that make up human beings. Each germ layer is responsible for each body part.

The outermost layer forms skin, nerves, and connective tissue that lie underneath the skin. The middle layer forms the circulatory system, muscle, bone, kidney and reproductive organs.

The innermost layer forms the tube with mucosa linings that makes up the gastrointestinal organs (gut system) and lungs.

Our organs are derived from these three layers. They are not connected to each other. They each have their own pathways. What we ingest is metabolized into small particles. These are absorbed into the blood through the lining of mucosa and circulate to all parts of the body. The liver controls the metabolism through the control of multiple hormone systems; the kidneys run the excretion system. The complexity of the kidney tubules is such that it does not let many large particles, like fat and protein, get excreted under normal conditions.

So do you see that the idea that when you use magic fat-melting creams or pills, the fat will come out through the urine can't be true.

It isn't biologically possible. **If a product advertises results in this way, you know that it's a scam.**

Normally, our kidneys can't excrete fat and protein in sufficiently large amounts to make it possible to lose weight. If a kidney is losing protein, it's a diseased kidney.

Dietary fat can be blocked so it doesn't get absorbed through the gut system, but if you do this you're also blocking the nutrients that get absorbed with the fat as well.

If some magic pill claims it can block your fat absorption in the gut system, you should know this is neither healthy nor biological and it will result in a loss of essential nutrients. When you lose the essential nutrients over a long period of time, your brain starts looking for it. You'll start craving more fatty food, and will end up gaining more weight in the long run. Also, as much as we want to lose fat, fat is an essential nutrient: you **must** have it in your body. If you starve your body of fat, your brain will crave it. Ever tried to fight a craving? It is not easy.

As fat is essential to the body, it can be synthesized from other macronutrients. The body will make it and manage to acquire it even if you try to block fat from your diet.

Fat is helpful and essential for our body because:
1. It keeps calories in storage.
2. It insulates our body from extreme temperatures.
3. It provides cushioning for our body and protects our internal organs.
4. We need it to produce hormones, vitamins, bile, and enzymes.
5. It is vital for the function of our nervous systems, needed by nerves to command signals that enable us to go about our daily lives.
6. It forms part of every single cell wall. So we cannot exist without fat.

Fat can't just melt away through the use of magical rays or the application of topical creams; the so-called melted fat has to somehow be discarded from the body. It can't just diffuse back into the large colon as excreta. It is also impossible for the kidney to excrete it out of the body as urine. Now there is liposuction, where the fat is sucked out with a suction device, but still the fact is that the fat can't return to the excretory system as one might think. (More about liposuction later in this book.)

Sometimes we wish so badly that something that lies just beneath the skin could somehow be taken out of the body by applying cream or light rays. It is wishful thinking, however, and marketers try to falsely grant this wish. But biologically, it doesn't work.

The other day I listened to an oxygenated water ad. Oxygen is desirable in our lives, but can we really further oxygenate water?

Water is made up of the molecule H2O; if the molecule is changed it won't be water anymore.

Just because regular water sounds boring, people start fancying vitamin infused water, fruit infused water, alkaline water — and now oxygenated water! But a chemist knows water can't be further oxygenated.

Oxygenated water sounds nice to drink, but can water be further oxygenated?

Bottom line: Don't be persuaded by marketing language.

Here I want you to pause and consider any diet techniques you've used in the past, or are using now, and get rid of anything that sounds logical but biologically won't work.

This is how we turn on the skinny switch: by getting rid of unhealthy weight loss practices. Now, you'll learn the basic biology of our body, and we will find the right weight-loss program for you. When you understand these basics, the rest is a piece of cake. In the future, no one will be able to persuade you with a quick-fix technique and you will save a lot of money, time and headaches.

HERE ARE SOME BASIC FACTS ABOUT HOW CALORIES WORK: UNDERSTANDING THE COMPOSITION OF OUR DIET.

Our diet consists of:

Calorie yielding macronutrients

Carbohydrates (aka carbs)

Examples: Rice, pasta, bread, potatoes, etc.

1 gram of carbohydrate gives you 4 calories.

Alcohol belongs to the carb group, but one gram of alcohol gives you 7 calories.

Protein

Examples: Chicken, pork, beef, seafood, pulses, tofu, etc.

1 gram of protein gives you 4 calories.

Fat

Examples: Butter, oil, lard, etc.

1 gram of fat gives you 9 calories.

Non-calorie yielding foods

Examples: Minerals, vitamins, electrolytes

This group does not provide calories, but these elements are essential for the metabolism.

There are three major macronutrients: Carbohydrates, Fats, and Proteins

1. CARBOHYDRATES

- Starches: potatoes, pasta, rice, etc.
- Fruit: apples, grapes, pears, etc.
- Fiber: this is the indigestible part of food
- Alcohol
- Legumes: peanuts, peas, beans, etc.
- Sugar

Carbohydrates are structurally made up of multiple sugar molecules. It is broken down to the smallest possible molecule in the gut before getting absorbed into the bloodstream. If a potato (polysaccharide) is ingested, it will be broken down by our digestive system in several steps. First we swallow and chew the potato; at this point it mixes with multiple digestive juices that break it down further into smaller and smaller pieces. Eventually, what began as a potato breaks down into a simple glucose molecule (monosaccharide). Now it gets absorbed into the bloodstream as sugar, while the fiber that remains in the gut is eventually excreted. This is known as a **slow-release sugar** because of so many steps needed to absorb it.

This process is different when you drink a sugary drink. Something like a sugary drink contains two molecules of glucose; this means it gets absorbed easily and instantly, without needing to go through the multi-step digestive process like the potato does. This is known as **fast-release sugar.**

Alcohol is another case altogether. When we drink alcohol, the alcoholic sugar (seven calories instead of four) is absorbed directly from our mouth, the oral cavity, as well as through the stomach. This is why we get tipsy even if we've had only a few sips. Alcoholic sugars are very rapidly absorbed into the blood stream. This is referred to as **super-fast and super-calorie yielding sugar**.

I've seen a billboard that advertises beer by saying "Beer isn't a sugar drink". This makes it sound like beer is better than a sugary drink as it seems it's not made of sugar.

If advertisers tell you it's a good idea to drink beer, even if you're overweight, you might be inclined to listen. The fact is though, that it's not a good idea. Beer is a super-fast and super-calorie yielding type of carbohydrate, and this kind of carb is definitely what you don't want to be consuming when you're trying to lose weight.

Marketing language can be persuasive, but the truth is that it's not a good idea to drink beer, which is an alcoholic beverage. Alcohol is the -OH (alcohol) form of sugar that is more toxic and destructive to the body, and it also yields more calories than regular sugar.

When you ingest carbohydrates, they break down to the smallest molecule (glucose) and are absorbed into the bloodstream.

The rate at which glucose increases in our blood determines how calories from that glucose will be utilized.

If glucose rises too quickly, in too-great amounts, it will stimulate a rapid insulin surge. The overwhelmed insulin will then store excessive glucose as fat, essentially acting to accumulate fat in the body. For example, if you drink sugary drinks throughout the day, you will be in fat-saving mode all the time.

A slow and steady rise of glucose will stimulate a slower insulin rise. In this case, the insulin is not overwhelmed and the excess glucose is used for several different things, including making glycogen, protein, and enzymes, as well as being used for other different bodily needs.

You can see how crucial it is to make informed decisions about the kinds of carb to consume. We'll discuss this further, later in the book.

2. FAT

- Animal fats
- Vegetable oil
- Fat in cheese and dairy products

Is fat good or bad? It's easy to find this confusing.

The truth is that fat can be either good or bad in our diets.

Fat is easy to eat and lends flavor to our food, and a small amount of fat is important, so we see that it's good to have fat in the diet.

On the other hand, fat is high in calories. It can quickly lead to weight gain, it can harden the arteries, and it can result in abnormal eating behavior, so we see that fat can also be a negative thing in the diet.

I use a minimal amount of fat in my diet. Don't block the fat in your stomach system by using so-called 'fat blocking' medicines. It will harm you more than you think.

⚡ FAT-ME-NOT TIPS

HOW TO USE MINIMAL FAT AND REDUCE YOUR FAT CALORIE INTAKE WITHOUT LIMITING FLAVOR OR TASTE:

1. Cook with vegetable oil at home: vegetable oil is cleaner and kinder to the arteries

2. Avoid using animal fat in cooking. The Fat-Me-Not Success Strategy Part III Chapter, later in the book, will go into deep-frying. I myself eat deep-fried food about four times a week without my arteries hardening, my cholesterol skyrocketing, or putting on any additional pounds.

3. When cooking, trim any fat off the meat. Avoid commercially ground meat. Ask the butcher to cut lean meat and grind it for you, or use a meat grinder at home. Only buy lean-cut meat from the store. Commercially ground meat has twice as much fat, or more, than lean ground meat.

4. At restaurants, ask for sauces or gravies on the side so that you don't end up eating all of the gravy. Gravy is basically nothing but flavored butter. You can eat some of the gravy, just not all of it. Sauce and gravy are for flavor and taste; we don't really need our food soaked in it.

5. Use an oil/butter sprayer for cooking and baking. One spray is only few calories while one teaspoon of oil/butter is around 100 calories, if not more. You can still use several sprays of butter on toast for a delicious flavor while leaving the fat calories behind.

6. When it comes to dairy products, choose a low-fat version.

WHAT YOU NEED TO KNOW ABOUT DIETARY FAT?

Usually dietary fat transforms into 'Acetyl CoA' in our body before turning into three different kinds of fat.

1. **Cholesterol**: This in turn makes hormones, which are a good thing. But if there is too much cholesterol, it may get deposited in your arteries and block blood flow.
2. **Triglycerides**: Triglycerides store energy for future use. If there is too much in storage, it becomes visible as lumpy spots on the body. Often if we find high triglycerides in our patients, we advise them to avoid sugars and carbohydrates, as the too-much too-fast rise in sugar may be what's causing them to store fat in this form.
3. **Phospholipids**: This is a kind of structural fat that aids in building individual cell walls.

Fat in our food is not a must-have; Acetyl CoA can be made from protein and carbohydrate.

Good essential fatty acid linoleic acid is important for keeping up our **fat burning metabolism**. In order to improve the production of the essential fatty acid linoleic acid in the body, we must:

1. Keep our blood sugar stable and lower, as high insulin impairs the production of this fatty acid.
2. Maintain an ample intake of magnesium, zinc, and B6.

Our metabolism is perfectly controlled by these little things. Limiting your diet, or depriving yourself of certain foods, will not create a perfect metabolism. For long-term effective weight-loss, dietary restriction just won't work.

As you see, fat is important part of our body composition. It is helpful to know how we can keep our body composition in perfect balance.

Taking multiple medications, especially steroids, can alter the shape and form of our bodies, including abnormal fat deposits, large buffalo humps on the neck, and round faces. Taking steroids results in these bodily distortions.

Sometimes, however, people have to take these medications to help them breath better or to relieve abdominal pain or joint pain, etc.

It is helpful to choose good kinds of fat, like omega 3 fatty acids, to aid in improving the shape of our body.

💡 FAT-ME-NOT TIPS

HOW TO IMPROVE THE SHAPE OF THE BODY:

1. Take omega 3 supplements or eat foods containing omega 3 such as fish and flaxseed.
2. Medium Chain Triglycerides (MCT) are abundant in coconut oil, chocolate, and palm oil. MCT is helpful for metabolizing fat and improving satiety. But too much of these can cause abdominal discomfort.
   I don't recommend adding coconut oil as daily supplement as it is high in calories. However, you can use it as a replacement for butter.
3. Lastly, get regular exercise

There are naturally good things in our daily diet, including fat. The important thing is to choose the **right portions** to create a balanced diet. This will keep our bodies' metabolism working efficiently.

3. PROTEIN

- Meat
- Eggs
- Legumes: beans and lentils
- Seafood
- Tofu
- Cheese (combined with fat)

Protein is a good nutrient; it is helpful for weight loss and is also useful for bodybuilding.

Protein is broken down into the smallest amino acid molecule before it is absorbed. Amino acids (protein) serve various purposes in our body. They build up the body and make enzymes, muscle, and other building blocks in the body. Our bodies have a protein storage pool; when you need the protein, it's taken from this pool. When the pool is diminished, it can be refilled for future use. Body has systematic control on supply and demand of protein stored as the protein pool.

As protein is a good nutrient, marketing labels on many products claim that their products are high in protein. This doesn't necessarily mean that protein bars, protein shakes, or protein drinks are better.

Let's take a look at how the body digests a regular piece of meat versus a protein powder drink.

Lets say that you have a 6-ounce steak and a protein drink, each of 350 calories. The two items contain the same number of calories and the same macronutrient.

When you eat a piece of steak, you enjoy the taste and feel satisfied as you eat a good meal. You also give the stomach system a workout by chewing (movement of the face muscles), swallowing (movement of the esophagus), mixing and churning of digestive juices in the stomach (movement of the stomach muscles), and secretion of bile acid and pancreatic juice (movement of the gall-bladder and pancreatic duct). The enzymes from the various digestive juices then break down the meat into the smallest molecule pieces called amino acids; those pieces are then absorbed into the bloodstream. By the time your meat is processed and absorbed, your stomach system has received a complete workout.

In contrast, when you drink a protein drink, you skip most of the stomach system workout. It is already in the form of an amino acid, so there's nothing to digest. Instead, the ready-made amino acids are directly absorbed into blood and there is no workout for the gut.

It is obviously not the same to eat a piece of meat or drink a protein shake, even though they have the same number of calories and same macronutrients. Thirty to thirty-five percent of the calories that you consume in real food will be burned by the workout of the gut. So eat real food. You get to eat real food while burning calories at the same time by making your gut work.

> *Bottom line: Your weight loss program should be based only on a real food diet not substitutes.*

So now what would you rather choose - a piece of real meat or a protein drink?

The next question that might come to mind is this: If a protein shake has all of the different essential amino acids complete within it, and a steak doesn't, then surely a steak can't be better?

There are only two super-essential amino acids; the rest can be made inside the body. These two essential amino acids are abundant in eggs and meat, for instance. If you aren't vegetarian, it is good for you to eat real meat and real food to give your gut a workout and speed up your metabolism, too.

Even if you're a vegetarian, if you eat dairy products and a variety of beans and legumes, this should be sufficient to acquire these essential amino acids.

Eat real food, including real meat, and give your gut a workout.

MARKETERS INFLATE CLAIMS TO SELL YOU STUFF

It's a known fact that garlic is good for lowering cholesterol. Marketers pick up this fact and make different types of garlic substitutes and sell them worldwide and make millions.

The fact that garlic helps to lower cholesterol is not sufficient to use it to treat a health condition like high cholesterol. Eating raw garlic may lower cholesterol 4-6% percent, but the amount you'd have to eat would result in the body reeking of garlic. Moreover the effect of the garlic is short-term; you would have to be on it for life in order to have that beneficial effect.

Usually when a diagnosis of high cholesterol is made, cholesterol is 30% or higher rather than 4-6% higher than normal range. Garlic may be good for cholesterol, but that on its own is not sufficient to treat a medical condition of high cholesterol.

This is true for most of the over-the-counter supplements such as Hoodia, green tea extract, guar gum, linoleic acid, chromium, garcinia cambogia, and green coffee beans. These are all ineffective for losing weight.

As yet, there are NO effective supplements on the market for losing weight.

PROTEIN IN THE BODY

Protein in the body is always changing; it is continually breaking down and producing protein substrates such as enzymes, hormones, collagen, and muscle. Constantly ongoing wear and tear is followed by constant repair and rebuilding.

This is a constant ongoing cycle; the protein pool is replenished with dietary protein constantly.

If protein intake is low, the turnover of the protein cycle is slow and sluggish. It uses less protein as we take in less.

If protein intake is high, the turnover of protein cycle is quicker; it makes and builds muscle, as well as other body needs. Excessive protein is excreted in the urine as nitrogen and creatinine.

Things like the degeneration process, aging process, sickness, physical and emotional stress, and rapid weight changes increase the demand for protein in the body. If not sufficiently replaced, the body loses its skeletal muscle, creating an aging-like appearance.

It is important to ingest enough protein daily to improve the metabolism and optimal body function.

> *Bottom line: Following a diet that deprives you of certain foods is never an option for effective weight loss.*

The micronutrients

MACRO MINERALS

1. Calcium
2. Chloride
3. Magnesium
4. Phosphorus
5. Potassium
6. Sodium

ORGANIC ACIDS

1. Acetic acid
2. Citric acid
3. Lactic acid
4. Malic acid
5. Choline
6. Taurine

TRACE MINERALS

1. Boron
2. Cobalt
3. Chromium
4. Copper
5. Fluoride
6. Iodine
7. Iron
8. Manganese
9. Molybdenum
10. Selenium
11. Zinc

MAGNESIUM IN THE BODY

Controlling the functions of cells, enzymes, and hormones is an important aspect to being able to keep our metabolisms running efficiently.

If there is insufficient magnesium in the body, we can suffer from chronic fatigue, painful muscle, overall weakness, and poor bone health.

But can we simply supplement magnesium with over the counter pills?

Magnesium can be ingested, but different dietary ingredients complicate its absorption into the body:

- Sugary drinks stop magnesium absorption
- Alcohol deprives the body of magnesium.
- A high starch diet stops the absorption of magnesium.
- A very low or a very high protein diet is not kind to magnesium absorption.
- Too much fat in the diet can cause magnesium pills to be a waste too.

Again, we see that the body is perfectly balanced. You cannot alter the balance by not eating certain foods and try to lose weight.

Weight loss has to happen while keeping this perfect balance approach.

Because of the complexity of magnesium absorption, an excess of magnesium can be harmful and life threatening. It's not recommended that you take extra magnesium as a regular supplement, though this is something you can discuss with your doctor, especially when you're experiencing symptoms. Magnesium levels can be measured, and make sure you keep a balanced diet to aid in its absorption.

CHROMIUM IN THE BODY

Chromium is a trace element. A chromium deficiency can cause insulin resistance, resulting in abnormal sugar levels, a decrease in lean body mass, an increase in fat mass, and increased body weight and neuropathy.

People on intermittent or long-term steroids, those who are under physical stress, and those who suffer an abnormal blood sugar condition may take chromium as a supplement.

Trace elements in our bodies are important for optimal metabolism, but these must also be in balance. Your body cannot have them in excess.

1. Iron deficiencies may cause cravings.
2. Zinc deficiencies may cause changes in taste.
3. Various vitamin B deficiencies can slow the metabolism; they are the co-factor of the metabolic pathway in our system.
4. Vitamin D deficiencies can cause musculoskeletal dysfunction.
5. Zinc supplementation, without copper, can create copper deficiencies.
6. Iron supplementation, without chromium, will cause chromium deficiencies.
7. Toxicity with cadmium, lead, mercury, and lithium can also alter other nutrients' bioavailability.

Antioxidants

- Alpha carotene
- Beta carotene
- Cryptoxanthin
- Lutein
- Lycopene
- Zeaxanthin

Vitamins

- Vitamin B complex,
- Vitamin B1 (thiamin)
- Vitamin B2 (riboflavin)
- Vitamin B3 (niacin)
- Vitamin B5 (pantothenic acid)
- Vitamin B7 (biotin)
- Vitamin B8 (ergadenylic acid)
- Vitamin B9 (folic acid)
- Vitamin B12 (cyanocobalamin)
- Group: pyridoxine, pyridoxal, pyridoxamine,
- Choline

All types of vitamin B are relatively safe as they are water-soluble and if consumed in excess can be excreted via the kidneys. Most types of vitamin B are important in the metabolic pathway; they are needed for perfect metabolism and for the body's fat-burning action. Vitamin B complex are generally responsible for skin and mucosal repair, nerve growth, and hair and nail growth.

Vitamin D

Vitamin D is important for musculoskeletal stability. Obese people tend to lack vitamin D, while around 50% of people 50 years and older also tend to be deficient. Individuals deficient in vitamin D often suffer from muscle weakness, bone frailty, unstable gait, and unexplained fatigue.

Antioxidants and vitamins

- Vitamin A (retinol)
- Vitamin C (ascorbic acid)
- Vitamin E (tocopherol)

Vitamins A, C, and E are well known for their antioxidant properties.

Antioxidants

Antioxidants are interesting nutrients. Our body deals daily with oxidative stress from chemicals trying to oxidize or react with our tissues. This can cause us to age, our bodies and organs to inflame, increase fat, and cause wear and tear of the body.

Anti-oxidants are the nutrients that help us block and clean up the destructive effects of this oxidative stress.

There are many antioxidants available; they vary in function, including when they work best in the body and which part of the body they work the best. In order to improve each and every part of our body, we need a variety of antioxidants.

Can too many antioxidants be harmful for the body?

Yes. Too much of an antioxidant can be harmful. Again, our bodies exist in a wonderful balance. The antioxidants must be in a good balance; there can't be too much or too little. Both extremes will cause an imbalance in the metabolism as well as tissue damage and inflammation.

Here are the best ways to supplement and optimize your diet using antioxidants. I don't suggest that you buy tons of antioxidants or supplement your daily diet with them.

Here is a list of food full of different antioxidants.

I want people to enjoy a variety of foods that are rich in antioxidants without worrying about an excess of antioxidants which can be harmful.

Antioxidant compounds	Foods containing high levels of these antioxidants
Carotenoids (carotenes, lutein, lycopene)	eggs, fruits, vegetables
Polyphenolic antioxidants (flavonoids, resveratrol)	chocolate, cinnamon, coffee, fruit, olive oil, oregano, soy, tea
Vitamin C (ascorbic acid)	fresh fruits, vegetables
Vitamin E (tocopherols, tocotrienols)	vegetable oils

Basically, meat, nuts, colorful vegetables, berries, chocolate, ginger, turmeric, dark green leafy vegetables, eggs, organ meat, fresh fruit, and even cooking oil are all good for us. They have positive nutritional value as well as antioxidants.

Bottom line: Eat real food and reap tons of benefits. It isn't harmful when you consume your nutrients in dietary form aka real food.

Don't Let Them Fool You

The metabolic control of the body is very complicated. There is no magic pill or substance to cure obesity. The best treatment is the maintenance of the overall balance.

Don't let weight-loss cure pills or over-the-counter supplements persuade you that it is the easy way. We don't need to be that desperate; we don't have to get blinded by these claims. Marketers don't know just how complex our bodies are. They only pull out one side of the story. For example, they might pick up on the idea that antioxidants are good. Then they advertise a bottle full of vitamin antioxidants and advise you to buy them at $20 per bottle. So we all go buy this bottle of vitamins, hoping that the pill can reverse all oxidative stress and thus rejuvenating, healing, and reducing inflammation in our body. The reality is that if you take too much of any antioxidant, you'll end up with side effects.

Though vitamin E is a very popular antioxidant that many people consume, vitamin E toxicity can cause muscle weakness, fatigue, nausea, diarrhea, and a tendency to bleed. Medscape ® reports that there are more than 60,000 cases of vitamin E toxicity reported annually to the US Poison Control Center.

Even though it is over-the-counter and it is just a vitamin, excess ingestion of vitamin E has the potential to be harmful.

In my daily practice, I have come across this problem many times. I now ask my patients to tell me about their over-the-counter medications when they see me at the clinic. People often consider over-the-counter (OTC) medications to be safe and neglect to mention them to their doctors.

As marketers who sell these OTC medicines do not know that the product can be harmful, they have no fear in claiming what they want to claim. You shouldn't fall victim to a lack of accurate information. Remember, marketers only know as much as you know; they don't know everything about the product. Marketers are only taught to tout the benefit of the product in their marketing language; this means the product will only come out as positive. All bad stuff is in the fine print that no one reads.

I know that these details of nutritional knowledge in this book may seem boring and too complex. My purpose here is to educate you enough that the marketing messages you are bombarded with every single day, won't mislead you.

What you need to do to lose weight in various conditions are in the Fat-Me-Not Success Strategy Part II Chapter; you will need to follow it. The knowledge you get in this chapter is beneficial knowledge. This way you know why you do what you do — it's not just because Dr. Nwe or Dr. Grewal says so.

What happens after you ingest food?

INTAKE SYSTEM

The foods we ingest are broken down into:

Free fatty acids (acetyl CoA) from fatty food

Amino acids from protein

Glucose from starches and carbohydrates

Then the nutrients are absorbed into the circulation crossing the intestine.

The circulation takes the nutrients to the different part of our body, including the brain, liver, and heart.

The various parts of the body then utilize the nutrients for energy which we call metabolism.

THE METABOLISM

Basically, metabolism is a complex function of the body; it builds what it needs, destroys what it doesn't, stores what it needs for the future, and transforms what it needs into the form it needs it in.

The metabolic process takes place in several parts of the body, mainly in the liver and muscle, but it happens in every cell.

The process is complex and requires many other micronutrients in order to optimize the process to produce energy. While producing the energy, it also utilizes the energy by itself.

THE STORAGE

What in the body needs glucose?

Every tissue in the body utilizes glucose for energy. It is essential for the brain and red blood cells (RBC) as both can only use glucose as source of energy. Brain cells can utilize ketone bodies, as a last desperate measure, only if the body is deprived of glucose. But Red Blood Cells, which carry oxygen to rest of the body, must have glucose.

So clearly we need to have glucose.

Now let's look at our body energy reserve. In what form our body stores energy producing nutrients?

1. **Small cap fund**

   Glycogen 200g; 800 *Cals* (*reflective of a 70kg man)
   Glycogen can be easily converted into Glucose. We will finish utilizing this source of energy in a few days, if we are in starvation mode.

2. **Mid cap fund**

   Protein 6,000g; 24,000 *Cals*

   When we run out of glucose and glycogen, we turn to body protein for energy. We can survive on this for a few weeks.

3. **Large cap fund**

   Fat 15,000g; 135,000 *Cals*

   We can survive on this for a few months.

HOW MANY CALORIES DO WE GET FROM 1 GRAM OF EACH FOOD GROUP?

Carbohydrate: 4 *Cals*/gram

Protein: 4 *Cals*/gram

Alcohol: 7 *Cals*/gram

Fat: 9 *Cals*/gram

It's not all math! There are other factors to it.

Excess carbs, sugars, and starches are converted to fat and stored for long-term use, while glycogen is stored for short-time use.

Excess fat is stored as fatty acids, fatty tissues, and lipids.

Protein can't be stored for long-term period after it is picked up by the protein pool. Protein pool provides short to medium term energy source. For long-term use, protein is transformed into fat and saved. Simply speaking, fat is the ultimate saving bank.

WHAT HAPPENS TO FOOD AFTER WE EAT?

There are three major food groups: carbohydrates, fat, and protein. They all are essential to our body. Thus any diets, that eliminate one of these food groups entirely, are not advisable and not safe and effective for weight loss.

Each food group generates ATP energy molecules for the body to use through different pathways.

Let's briefly talk about how these foods break down (degrade).

Carbohydrates break down to
1. Glucose: for instant energy
2. Glycogen: for energy reserves, to maintain the blood glucose level between meals

Glycogen is stored in the liver and muscle and can store up to 800 Cals. The glycogen store constantly replenishes as soon as we use it. During starvation, the brain can use this glycogen storage for few days to function.

Fat breaks down to free fatty acids. These bind with albumin in the blood and are transported to cells. They also bind with oxides for energy (ATP). But the brain and RBC can't utilize free fatty acids.

The liver can metabolize free fatty acids into ketone bodies. The ketone bodies are utilized by muscle for energy and by the brain during starvation if glucose is not available.

Protein breaks down into amino acids. Amino acids are building blocks of the body protein and are precursors for many other physiologically important compounds, including neurotransmitters and hormones. Protein is not a major source of energy like glucose and fat. It is mainly used as energy to bridge between the carbohydrate and fat energy gap. The body takes approximately two weeks to start utilizing the fat as a major energy source after depleting the carbohydrate energy source. If we have sufficient energy from carbohydrates and fat, the protein is mainly used for repair and the forming the body protein (e.g., hormones and enzymes).

THE TRANSFER OF NUTRIENTS FROM ONE PART TO ANOTHER

The food and the drink that we consume through the mouth is digested by various parts of intestine using hormones and enzymes. Then it crosses the membranes from gut to capillaries (vessels) and into the main bloodstream to the organs (such as the liver, kidneys, and muscles).

It involves a special transport system for different nutrients with various different mechanisms under the control of hormones and chemicals in our body. All you need to understand is that foods diffuse from one place to another as a very small, invisible particle. Undigested and large residues are waste products and are excreted.

THE EXCRETION SYSTEM

The body excretes via the following organs:

1. The liver is responsible for the excretion of ammonia (the waste product of protein) by transforming it to urea, and also excretion of fat into bile in the gut.
2. Bile acid and bile salt are excreted as a bilirubin by-product of red blood cells.

3. The kidneys excrete excess water, urea, nitrogen, uric acid, and ammonia.
4. The bowels excrete solid waste products from unwanted fats, fibers, water, gases (nitrogen and sulfide), and even excess bacteria.
5. Unwanted salt and water are excreted through the skin via the sweat.
6. The lungs expel unwanted gases such as carbon dioxide.

Now you understand how the body processes our food. Now you can see the following myths for what they really are.

Myth #1

If you do not eat, you will lose weight

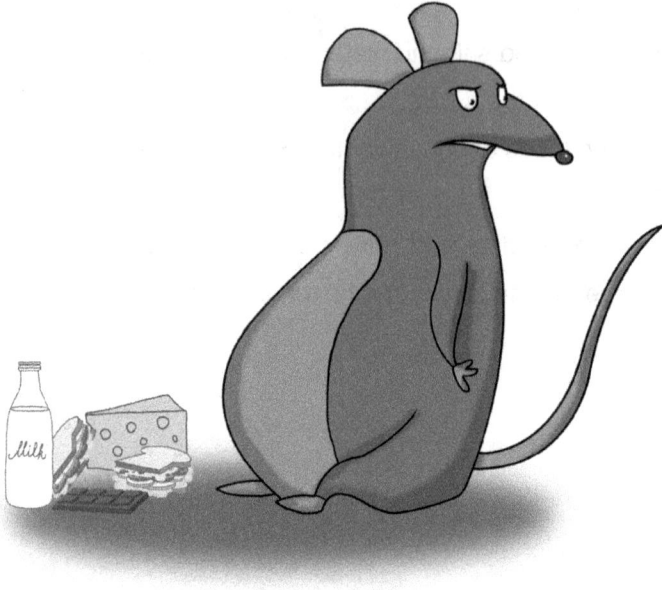

This is wrong.

Suppose you don't eat for several hours, or even for days. Your body will switch on the Starvation Mode. This will cut down your calorie expenditure to less than 40% and also promote fat storage by triggering the fat-saving mechanism.

This is why, when we're hungry, we can't focus, think, do chores, or do exercise.

It is proven that if children eat breakfast regularly, their academic and physical performance is better than that of a child who doesn't eat breakfast.

If you don't eat you are defeating the purpose of losing weight.

Myth #2

If you only eat once a day, you will lose weight

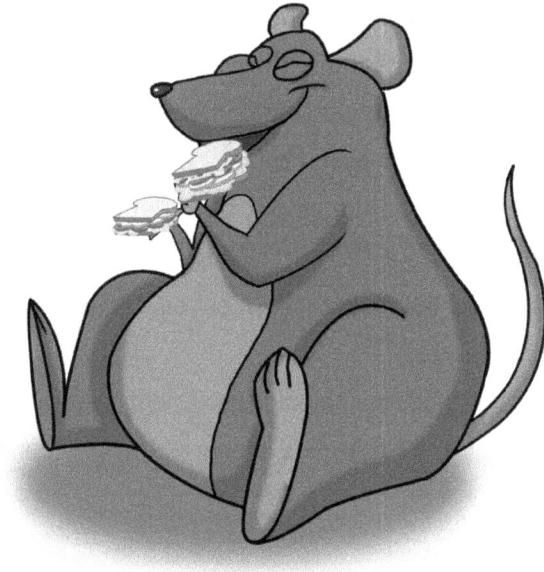

This is wrong. But many of us still do it.

If you habitually do not eat every 4-6 hours while awake, your body goes into Starvation Mode and starts storing fat, shutting down the energy/calorie spending process. Your metabolic rate will go down and you will spend fewer calories.

If you commonly skip breakfast, and have lunch at noon, you may be creating a starvation mode.

The most calories spent in our body are a result of the stomach, not the heart, brain, skin, or urinary systems. The stomach and intestines spend a whopping 35% of the calories we take in every day.

So by eating once a day you are not giving a good workout to your stomach system. You're not maximizing your calorie spending for the best weight-loss result.

Let's say you eat 1500 *Cals* per day. If you eat frequently, about 500 Calories will be spent by your stomach workout. To spend 500 calories, you have to work out hard at the gym i.e. more than 2-3 hours as an average woman. Burning these number of calories can be achieved more simply by eating frequently.

What's the right thing to do?

Eat frequently 4- 5 times per day. I let my very obese patients eat about 6-8 times a day, as initially they need more calories and they feel hungry. But making them eat so frequently also helps them burn more calories.

Eat a variety of foods, including fruit, meat, vegetables, and even fat.

Eat real food. Choose real piece of meat rather than a protein drink or bar.

Myth #3

Diet sugar and diet drinks are good for losing weight

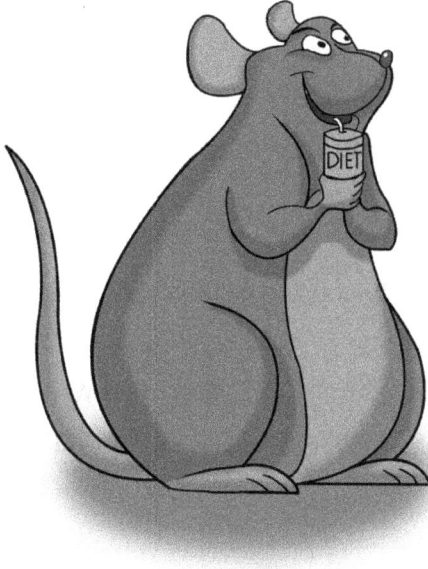

Diet sugar is an anti-nutrient. It works against nutrients. Replacing sugar with artificial sweetener is one of the worst things that happened to our food industry. Mass adoption of wrong habit of drinking diet drinks and using artificial sweeteners is already widespread. These things happen because the lack of scientific research. We learn things backward. Instead of learning the right way and putting it into action, we act and then realize it is not right.

People think of logic and apply logic to the human body, when the human body is biological and works differently than logic.

The logic is that if sugar gives unwanted calories but we want a sweet taste, we should replace it with something that gives us the taste but not the calories. Looks like a win-win logic.

But the human body is biological. The brain is super smart and remembers the sweetness and calories together. When it gets only sweetness without the calories, it looks for the calories even more. It makes you crave junk food because you cannot replace breads and cakes with artificial stuff. You can't fool the brain.

There are many other side effects that accompany artificial sweeteners, including feeling dizzy, headaches, and fogginess of the brain.

So it is not right to replace sugar with artificial sweeteners. Instead, portion your sugary drinks to Fat-Me-Not levels and we will discuss that later in the book. That is what we have done in the SlimPlate System drink cups also. So you can enjoy the real sugar but in right amount.

Myth #4

Fast food is bad, but fine dining is okay

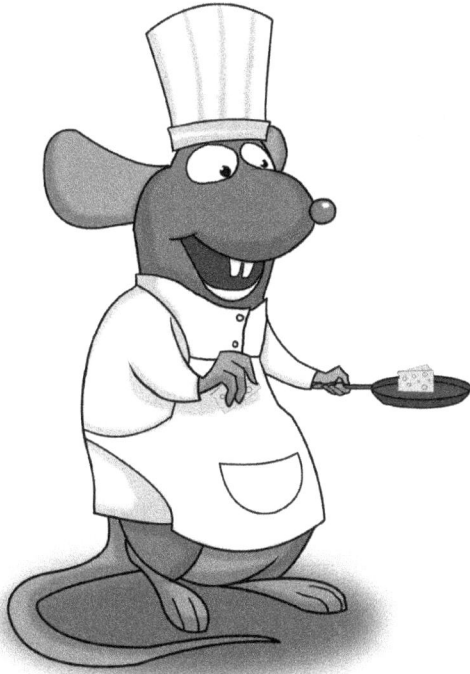

The question here is if the restaurant food is healthier than the fast food?

I want to share an experience where I had a great dinner, freshly prepared by a famous chef right in front of us. I was with eight other physicians at a special dinner that was prepared live right in front of us.

The event was wonderful. The meal was phenomenal.

The meal was served like this:

Shrimp scampi puff (appetizer, one small piece each)

Salad with balsamic vinegar dressing (small green salad with goat cheese, dried raspberries, and nuts)

Roasted beef with lobster stuffing (measuring half the size of your palm)

Potato side dish (two finger-long sized pieces)

Sautéed asparagus side dish (5-6 slender pieces)

Banana in brown sauce with a small scoop of ice cream; a thin slice of pound cake (regular portion)

A glass of wine

It was a wonderful meal, portioned just right without being excessive. Usually I would not be thinking that this was an unhealthy meal, if it was not cooked in front of me.

Everything was cooked right in front of us so I saw all the ingredients used. The art and skill of the chef was amazing. But what was going through my mind was "nine of us shared seven sticks of butter, four large blocks of cream cheese, and a bowl of clarified butter over a two and half hour meal?"

I can't believe I ate nearly a stick of butter and half of a large block of cream cheese in one meal.

While I do appreciate the time, the dinner, and the chef, I would not repeat the meal again.

The thought of cholesterol plaques blocking my arteries kept bouncing through my head.

I discovered the following from this wonderful dinner:

Chefs are excellent at preparing food but they may not have the nutritional knowledge.

A chef's main focus is to make the food taste better, not necessarily to make it healthier.

Expensive upscale restaurants, compared to fast food joints, do not necessarily mean the food is healthier.

While we avoid fast food chains when trying to eat healthy, it's easy to end up like me in the above situation.

Cook healthily at home. Don't use butter or similar fats for cooking a meal; use a non-butter spread. I do not believe that using so much butter and cream cheese was necessary for that wonderful meal. I recreated the meal without using the butter and cream cheese. I substituted olive oil and boiled low-fat milk, which resulted in a comparable taste and a greater health benefit.

If you are already in a restaurant, ask for your gravy or sauce to be put on the side so that you don't have to eat it all. That is where most of the fat and grease is.

Avoid restaurants that cook with butter and cream cheese, or at least don't let these restaurant dinners be a regular occurrence.

Myth #5

Eating salad and grilled chicken is the way to go for weight loss

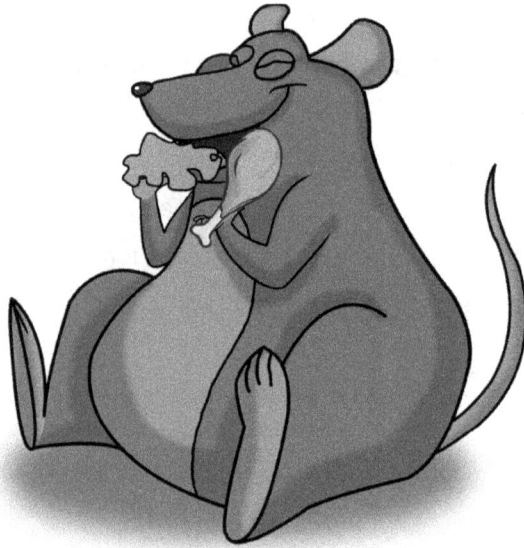

This is wrong.

As you know by now, eating grilled chicken and raw salad is not the way to go for weight loss. We need a balanced diet; vegetables, meat, and starch are all needed. Grilled is good, but there is nothing wrong with deep-fried or stir-fried or curry or any other style. (I will teach you how to deep-fry food and feel calories-careless in your mind).

The more variety of food, the better it is.

Why cut starch when you're trying to lose weight? You don't need to cut out carbs for weight loss. You can eat starches; all you need to do is keep the portions correct.

There is nothing wrong with eating fruit, chips, french fries, or popcorn for snacks as long as you maintain the portion in the snack bowl. For those using the SlimPlate system, the fruit saucer is the correct portion. If you don't, just a handful of snacks is the right portion.

Eat many varieties of food and enjoy them.

You can eat anything in the world (except diet sugar), but you must portion it right.

This includes cake, cookies, and anything else — you just have to portion them. Some health gurus argue that sweets are a taboo in weight loss diets. I will explain in a later chapter how one can go out of control, making it difficult to portion processed sweet foods and how these sweet cravings happen.

Rest assured, if you follow the instruction in this book on how to eat sweets (mentioned in a later chapter) and portion them correctly, you can eat any sweet you like. The fact is that food craving and binging comes from the negative impact of deprivation and an unbalance diet. When you are on a balanced diet, you do not have to fear these abnormal eating behaviors.

Myth #6

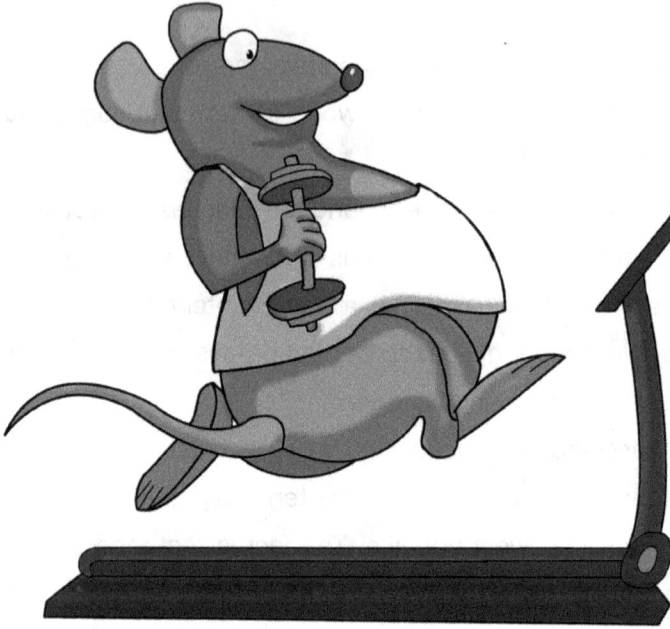

If you cannot exercise, you will not lose weight. Who said that?

People only see the physical workout. The major workout is not physical; there are gut workouts too – when we digest our food.

If you eat the right portions, at right time with real food, this will do the workout for you. It will improve your metabolism, send the right signal to the brain via Fat-Me-Not gut hormones and bacteria, and send down the Fat-Me-Not signals and switch you from Fat-Me-Yes cycle to Fat-Me-Not cycle where it is much easier to maintain weight. More about these cycles in later chapter.

Don't give up or think that if you can't do exercise, that you're supposed to be fat.

By now you know the body works in balance.

I have many patients, who have successfully changed their diet to Fat-Me-Not and able to lose weight. Many of them couldn't exercise because of their age or disabilities.

Don't give up! Break this myth of impossibility.

Myth #7

Eating carbs will make you fat

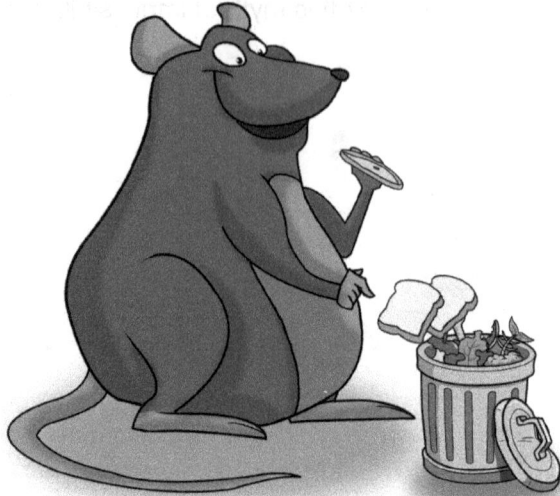

The carbohydrate content of a meal should be around 40-65% of your daily calories. Bread, rice, pasta, and potatoes are all okay to eat.

Choose to eat more unrefined (wholegrain) portion each time.

Don't eat six sandwiches or three pancakes or four slices of toast or an entire watermelon. These aren't the right portions.

Eat unrefined versions of carbohydrates mixed with fiber; these are good kinds of carbs. If you eat bread or rice or pasta, mix it with vegetables; combine bread with tomato, mushroom, onion, or pickle to make a sandwich; and add vegetables to your pasta. Choose the wholegrain version of bread or pasta.

High carb diets filled with complex carbohydrates like wholegrain starches and high fiber are desirable for weight loss.

What you should avoid is highly processed carbs like high fructose corn syrup, high sugar drinks, and cakes and pastries with high sugar or fructose corn syrup.

Don't give up carbs in order to lose weight; this will only create a disaster in your body. Remember the wonders of balance. We have to be in balance for maximum weight loss and long-term weight loss.

Here I need to stress that long-term weight loss does not mean slow weight loss; it only means effective weight loss that lasts!

I learnt the importance of emphasizing that lasting weight loss is not a slow process, from a patient of mine. I always want long-term success for my patients from the beginning. She kept telling me that she needed to lose forty pounds before her wedding in six months. She asked me if this was possible.

I thought she would lose weight in a timely fashion. She then asked me if there was a program that would help her lose weight faster.

Then I realized that as I had mentioned long-term success repeatedly, she thought I was putting her on a slower weight-loss program.

Finally understanding her, I explained that she would lose weight at a good pace and that the result would be long-lasting.

Long-term weight loss doesn't sacrifice the effectiveness of initial weight loss.

Myth #8

Switch from caffeinated to decaffeinated to lose weight

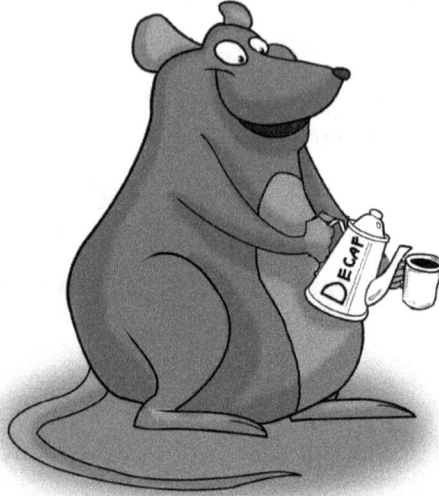

Caffeinated drinks, like coffee or tea, are okay to drink in correct portions. You don't need to change to decaffeinated as caffeine actually helps increase metabolism a little bit.

The reason we portion the drink is to limit the sugar content to avoid triggering fat-saving mode. If you like black coffee without sugar, you should drink a few drinks a day.

The only concern with the caffeine is that it can increase heart rate and heart irregularity and may increase blood pressure if you drink too much.

If one to three cups of black coffee floats your boat, then that's what you should do.

Myth #9

Eating sweets, desserts, and chocolate are no-nos for weight loss

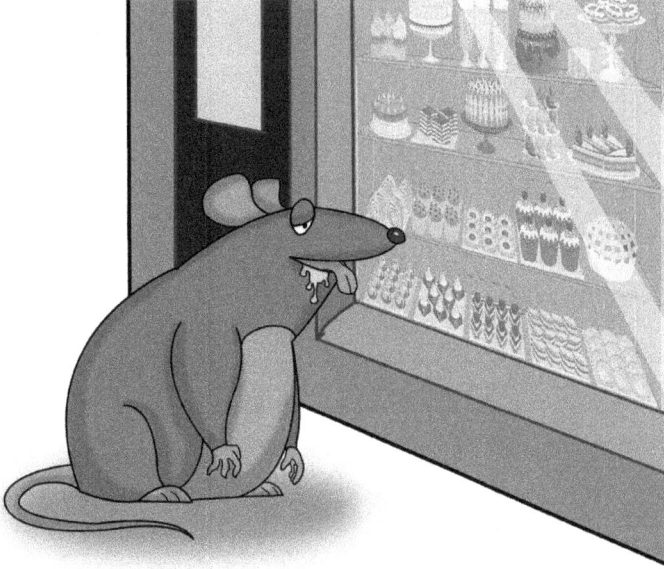

No sweets = No life.

You don't have to take away every good thing from your diet. Just portion them to the right size and right time.

You can't eat a large pie to replace dinner, just as you can't eat a bowl of ice cream to replace your lunch.

Sweets and desserts are for savoring, not for replacing the meal. You will never be satisfied if you eat sweets for a meal. This will disturb the balance of our metabolism.

Eat sweets as dessert and keep the portion as allowed. (You can download and refer to the free SlimPlate System mobile app for right chocolate and snacks portions.)

Myth #10

Obesity is healthy and there is nothing wrong with it

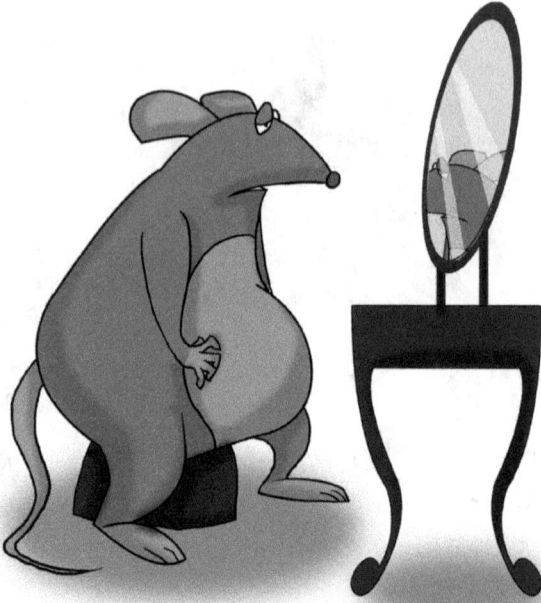

Obesity is not normal and not healthy. Obesity is a killing disease. In the next chapter we talk about real stories that explain how obesity destroys our lives and health.

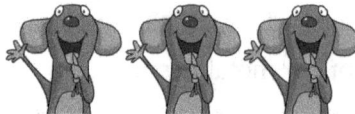

Chapter 3
The Killing Machine

How Obesity Can Sabotage Your Health and Life?

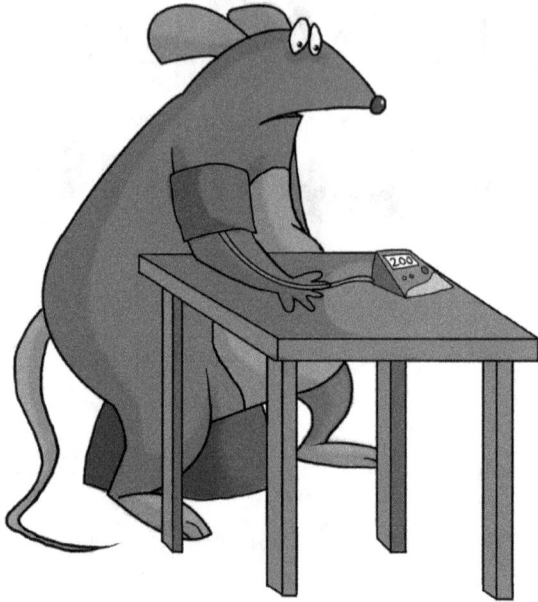

High blood pressure is twice as common in people who are obese or overweight

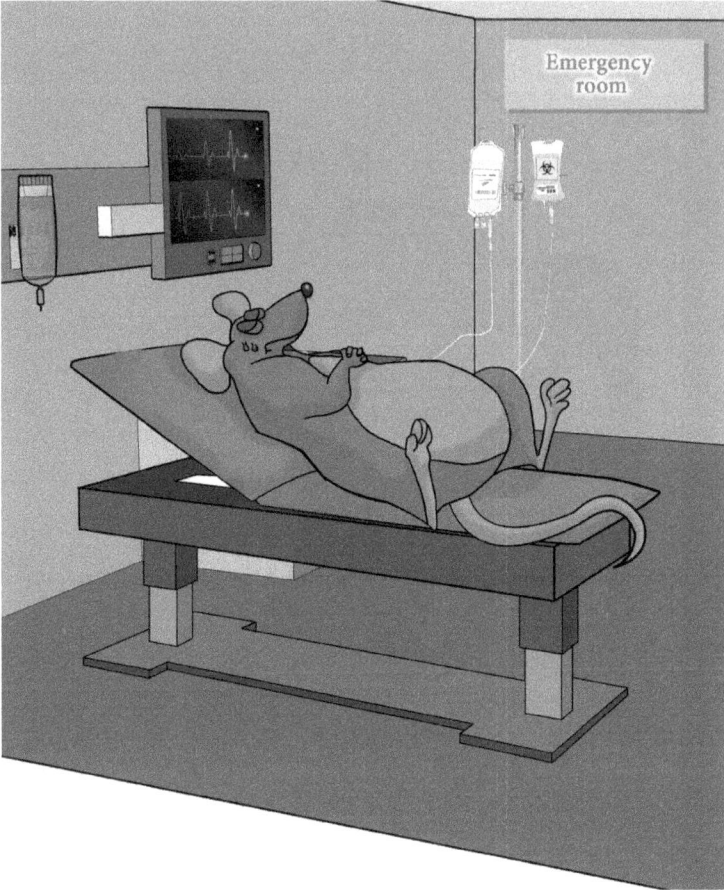

Obesity increases the risk of heart attacks by 60%

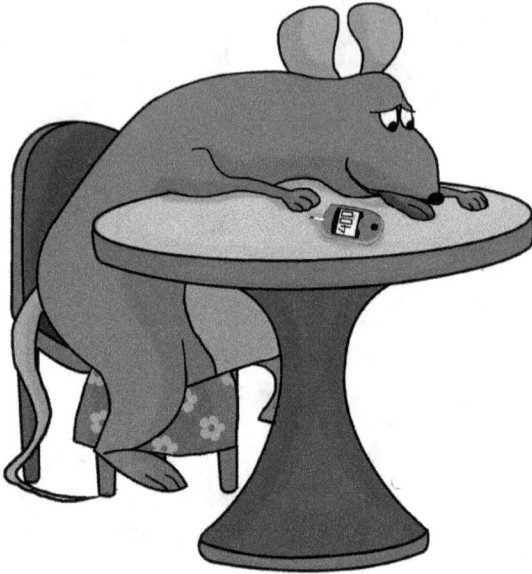

Eighty percent of patients with diabetes are obese or overweight

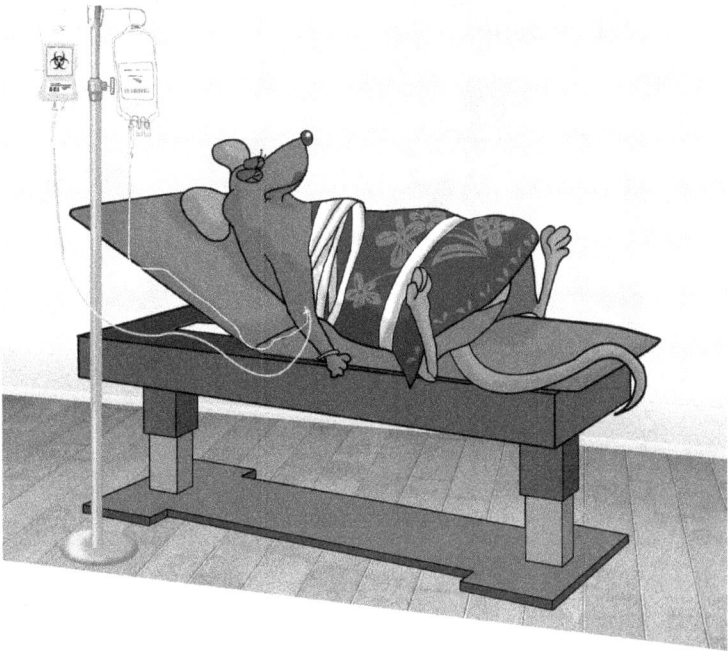

Obesity increases the risk of certain types of cancer

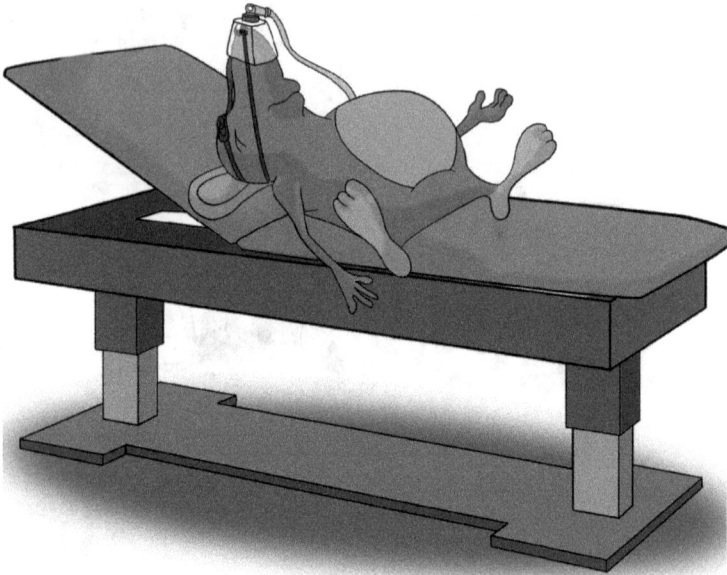

Obesity doubles the chance of getting sleep apnea

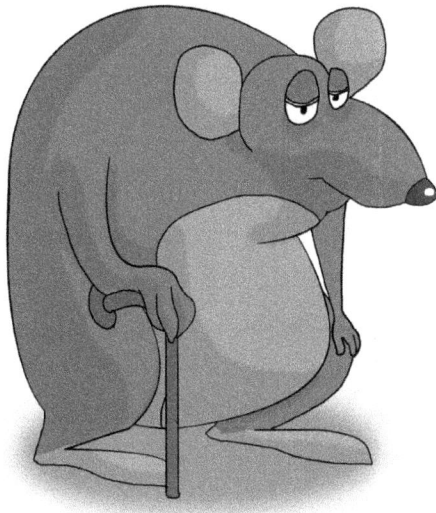

Obesity can increase the risk of joint pains by 60%

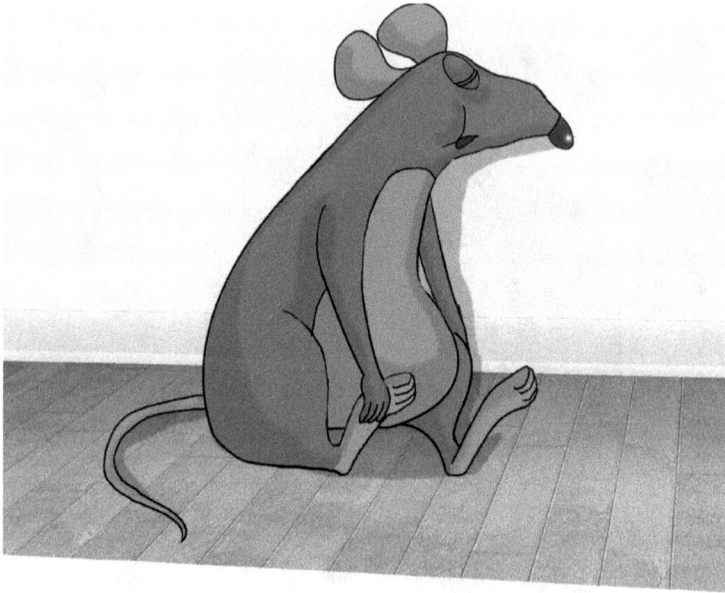

Obesity can reduce your overall well-being and cause you continual
fatigue

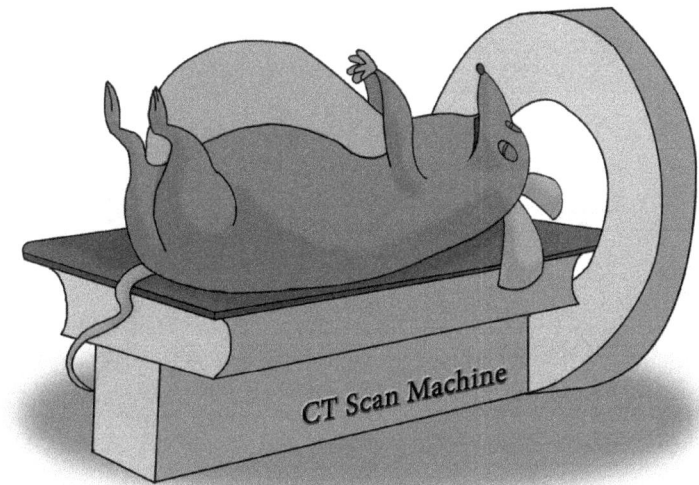

CT Scan Department

CT Scan Machine

Obesity can make it difficult to detect diseases

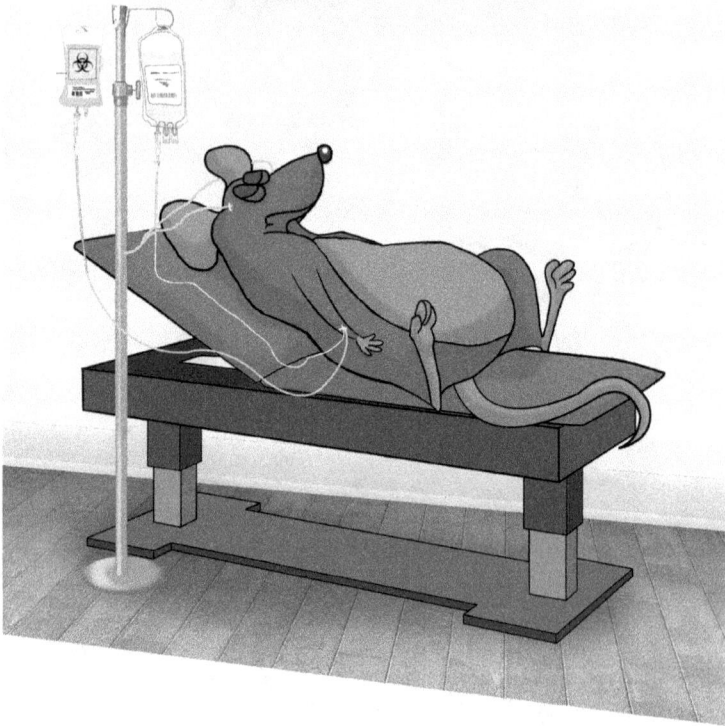

Obesity can increase the risk of stroke

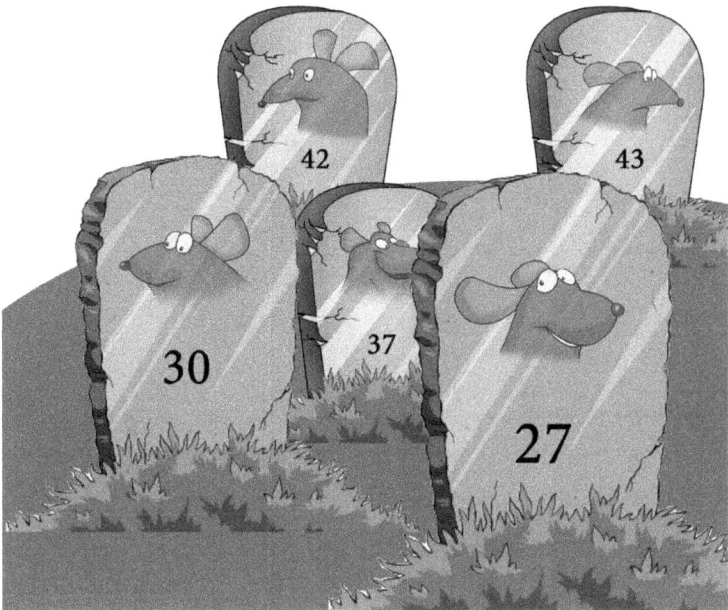

Obesity increases the risk of premature death

Obesity kills: It is not only a personal concern but a public concern

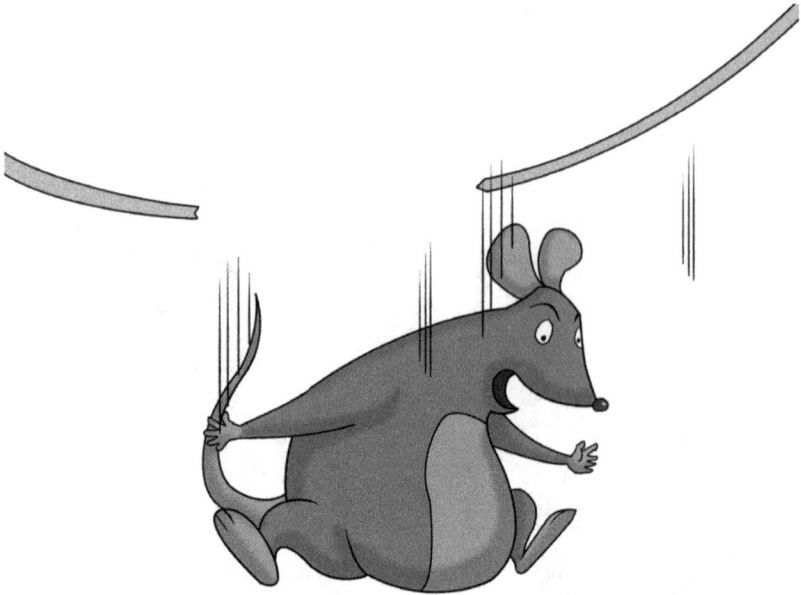

I read about the conflict between Governor Christie and Dr. Mariano. I don't want to judge who is right or wrong, but I'd like to take a moment to express my concern.

Your personal appearance is your concern, but obesity isn't personal any more. It is a health concern, which makes it a doctor's concern as they must take their patients' best interests into consideration. If a patient is at an unhealthy weight, it's almost impossible during a doctor's consultation not to discuss the need for weight management.

Obesity kills!

We lose many people at young ages to obesity — nineteen-year-olds, thirty-seven-year-olds, forty-three-year-olds and more. Sometimes, obesity does not kill the body outright, but slowly destroys different parts of the body until the whole body ultimately fails and dies. Carrying one hundred extra pounds means that with each passing day knees, hips, ankles, pancreas, heart, brain, kidneys, etc. are all wearing out at quadruple the speed. This extra weight also makes it difficult to reach down to the lower part of the body, meaning that there is an increased risk of lower extremity infection, which can result in hospitalization, infection, and can make people homebound.

I strongly agree with Dr. Marino about one thing: obesity is not a laughing matter.

The main cause of the obesity epidemic is a lack of awareness and a lack of education about the problem. Strangely enough, the United States has the largest obesity population in the world. In the US, the obesity rate is 30.6%; in Japan it's 3.2%; Canada 14.3%; France 9.4%, and Italy 8.4%.

Once a personal concern, Obesity is now a national concern.

I used to hear people being awed about how great Americans are. They'd mention American football and traditional American Thanksgivings, but now, instead of comments about how great Americans are; I hear questions about what's going on with our country. A well-travelled, nationally known executive pointed out that Americans are big, wondering why this was so.

There are many reasons why Americans are so big. The main reason is that we can't accept when people ask for help, or indeed ask for help ourselves; we struggle to commit to improve ourselves;

and we fail to offer support, thinking that it's someone else's personal issue and it's not our place to interfere.

When a large company employer wanted to buy weight-loss portion control plates for their employees in order to promote better health and physical fitness, the employer was reminded by his advisor that the employees' obesity was their own personal issue.

It is not okay to be obese. It is a health risk. Obesity can snatch you away from your loved ones. Obesity can destroy your mind, body and spirit if you don't fight it.

Don't let yourself be misinformed; obesity and health can't coexist.

In the media, people say that there is nothing wrong with being obese. Some people say that it is harmless, that those concerned about obesity is another attempt to get media attention. But I think that acting in this manner is irresponsible, as it is misleading and represents obesity incorrectly to the general public as being safe.

In the next chapter we will talk about how to get the right mindset to lose weight. It is important to have the right mindset because that is what you need to sustain a weight loss effort.

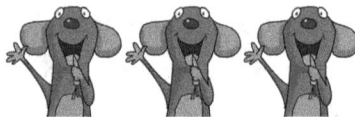

Chapter 4
Turn Off The Fat Switch

Get Ready to Lose Weight with the Right Perception

1. *Obesity is a disease; it needs to be treated appropriately.*

2. *Just because insurance may not cover treatment does not mean that obesity is not serious enough to be treated.*

3. *The only way to lose weight is to change your lifestyle long-term, including diet, physical activity, and eating behavior. This must continue even after weight loss surgery, if done.*

4. *Choose the weight loss plan that works well with your life in order to adhere to it for a lifetime.*

5. *Anything that claims to promote weight loss but that you cannot sustain for a lifetime will only destroy your weight control system, resulting in additional rebound weight gain.*

6. *The only way to lose weight is to eat real food.*

7. *Strenuous workouts are not necessary to lose weight.*

8. *You must drink water regularly to quench your thirst and keep hydrated; this will automatically work to cleanse and detox you.*

9. *Many medications may prevent you from losing weight.*

10. *Give up artificial and natural sweeteners.*

Obesity is a disease; it needs to be treated appropriately

The most important initial step to successful weight loss is changing one's perception.

In a metropolitan hospital in 2013, a doctor was taking care of a patient in a hospital. The patient had been in the hospital three times in the preceding three months, and he asked the doctor what the real problem with him was.

The patient was admitted with difficulty breathing and respiratory failure. He weighed 350 pounds, but he was neither a smoker nor an asthmatic.

He said, "Doctor, I don't smoke. I don't work in a chemical plant, or in any kind of a dusty environment. Why is my breathing so bad? Tell me what I can do to improve it."

The doctor explained that the patient had a condition called "Obesity Hypoventilation Syndrome". He explained to the patient that his weight is crushing his chest and preventing his lungs from expanding. Obesity Hypoventilation Syndrome, the doctor explained, is a condition where there is an excess of fat in the body, and this begins to suffocate the person — they are unable to breathe. He told the patient that losing weight could cure this condition.

A few days later, the doctor received a letter detailing a complaint that the patient had filed against him. The patient argued that the doctor had no idea about his "disease", instead blaming it on his "condition" that is obesity. He requested to be switched under care of a different doctor with more knowledge who might be able to correctly identify the patient's disease.

Obesity is a disease. Among other things, it disrupts bodily functions. Unfortunately, many people think of obesity as a condition, meaning that many may be at risk without ever thinking of themselves as having an illness.

The following chapters explain how obesity disrupts the body, just like any other disease.

Just because health insurance may not cover treatment does not mean that Obesity is not serious enough to be treated

There are multiple reasons why health insurance plans do not cover obesity.

In the last fifty years, there has been a fairly sudden rise in obesity rates. However, this rise has been peaking in the years following 1990, meaning that the disease is both relatively new and beginning to draw more notice.

Obesity is also perceived differently; more than half of overweight people think that they are at an acceptable weight. Many obese individuals are aware that their weight is above normal; yet do not believe that it is at an unhealthy level. This results in a widespread confusion in which obesity is not perceived as a disease that needs to be treated.

Health plans will have to shell out money to treat obesity. Costs for weight management treatments and services have increased by 30% in a short time. There is a "don't ask, don't give" policy.

There is also a lack of a standard treatment guideline to treat obesity. It wasn't until relatively recently, in 2013, that the American Medical Association declared obesity to be a disease; the American College of Cardiology/American Heart Association and the Obesity Society only established obesity guidelines in November 2013.

Meanwhile, weight management service providers still number less than a few thousand to date. So there is a shortage of treatment providers also.

This book aims to establish that it is our own responsibility to keep our own weight in check. In order to improve our own health, we must keep our weight under control. The latest improvements in obesity and weight management policies, procedures, and guidelines are the reasons to be hopeful for the future, but ultimately we are responsible for reaching and maintaining a healthy weight ourselves.

Weight loss dieting is a not a short-term plan. The only way to lose weight is to change your lifestyle long-term, including diet, physical activity, and eating behavior. This must continue even after weight loss surgery, if it is done.

There is so much information available that it is easy to be confused by conflicting data, misinformation, and marketers-directed information.

What are you going to go through to correctly lose weight? Remember, logic does not work when it comes to losing weight; it has to be biologically correct.

Here is what successful weight loss plans feature, in a very simple way.

Everyone should know that the definition of success in weight loss is not just losing the weight but also being able to keep that weight off long-term. There are three criteria that must be met for any diet plan to be successful.

A diet has to be easy to do. If it is not easy to do, it cannot be sustained for long periods and rebound weight gain is inevitable.

For a diet to be successful, it must use real food. Protein shakes, bars, and frozen foods are not our natural foods; any diet relying on these foods will eventually fail. Our brains are designed to seek real food; trust me, it will.

A good diet plan should change behavior and eating habits. It is our old habits that cause weight gain so until those habits are gone – and I mean gone forever – we cannot escape from rebound weight gain.

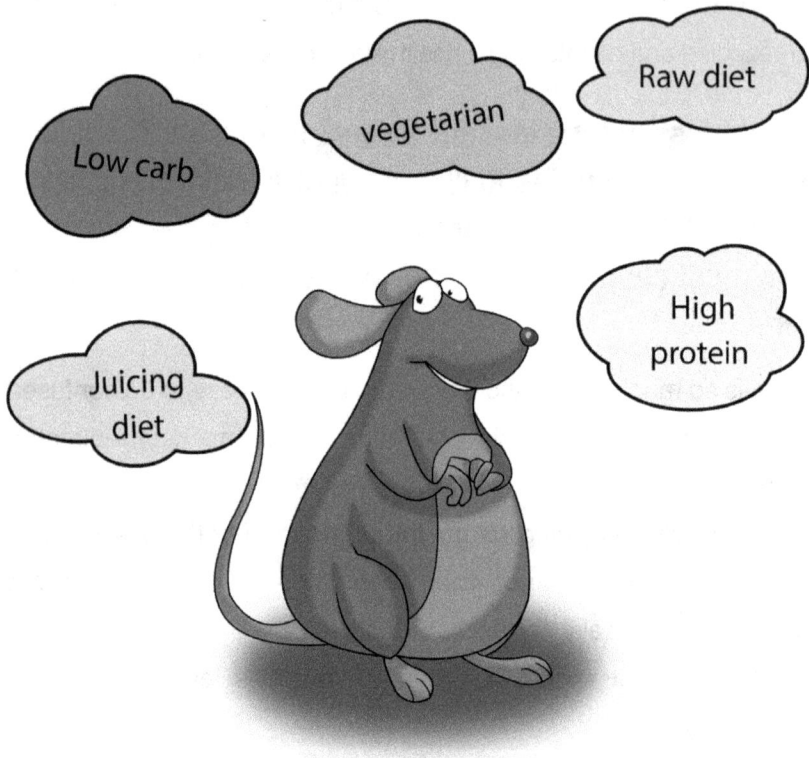

The only way to lose weight is changing the long-term life style of diet, physical activity and eating behavior

There are multiple diets plans out there.

Frozen diets

Raw diets

Juicing diets

No carb diets

Low calorie diets

These diets are all wrong; you can't eat raw or frozen food for life. It is equally impossible to sustain a diet consisting of juices, no carbs, or low calories. When the hype is over, rebound weight gain will hit you and pack even more pounds than before. Ultimately, you will end up bigger in size and smaller in confidence, making it much more difficult to lose weight again.

Many times my patients have come to me, excited, and told me, "Doctor, I lost seven pounds with this juicing diet I started three weeks ago."

I tell them do not do it, that it will not last and they will gain the weight back in no time.

I sometime feel like a parent who has had to put a harsh stop to their kid's newfound puppy love.

But if I do not do it, then the next time I see my patients, they are bigger in body and smaller in self-esteem.

I have yet to see a person who has successfully kept weight off for very long as a result of these temporary diets.

Again and again, my patients tell me: "I didn't watch my diet like before and it all came back."

Successful diets do not have to be watched daily. You must turn it into a habit that you can keep going for life.

Choose the weight loss plan that works well with your life in order to adhere to it for a lifetime.

If you're not vegetarian, don't plan to become one.

If you enjoy steak, don't plan to get rid of steak and only eat chicken.

If you are an Italian, eat like an Italian.

If you are an Asian, eat like an Asian.

If you are an American, eat like an American.

You can modify the food you grew up eating in order to develop the healthy habits but you cannot change the fundamental ingredients because you grew up eating those ingredients.

Anything that claims to promote weight loss, but that you cannot sustain for a lifetime will only destroy your weight control system, resulting in additional weight gain

If a diet plan doesn't meet the above three criteria, do not start it; it will destroy the weight control signals in your body. I will explain the weight control signals in a later chapter.

One of my obese patients told me that she did not want to lose weight. She was not kidding.

She explained, "I don't want to try to lose weight any longer because I have tried to lose weight several times. And every time I lost weight, I gained much more back later. I am currently at 289 pounds. If I had never tried to lose weight before, I could have weighed less than 289 pounds now."

Surprisingly, I agreed with her because I know she was right.

Every time we alter the weight control signals in our own body, there are consequences. If the change that you make isn't for the long-term, your body will rebound.

The only way to lose weight is to eat real food

Don't look for non-biological ways to shed weight. I have already explained why non-biological ways are not going to keep your body lean.

Eat real food. Buy healthier versions of the food you enjoy. Eat in portions. Use effective portion control methods such as the SlimPlate System. Enjoy different varieties of food (different vegetables, meat, starches, fruits, nuts, and snacks).

Balanced nutrition and balanced conditions (for example, staying healthy, not stressed, not sleep deprived, and keeping a hormonal balance) in the body results in best metabolism and best weight loss.

Strenuous workouts are not necessary to lose weight

Many of my patients can't get heavily involved in an activity when they first try to lose weight. But they lose weight.

The reality is many of obese people can't work out like the model running on the treadmill in television commercials.

These ads show people motivated to exercise, and projects the idealization of the results you can get from the machine or the product they advertise.

If I were to ask my patients to do these strenuous exercises in order to lose weight, I can say that 100% of people would quit by day two, or they would injure their joints and muscles, perhaps even damaging their backs.

Don't be discouraged by your physical limitations and don't lose the confidence to lose weight effectively.

Exercise comes after, once you lose some weight and you are physically able to do it. Your body will tell you when you are able to do the physical activity. You won't be able to do it on day one, but after you lose weight you will be able to.

Thirty minutes of exercise for the average person spends about 120 calories (it is more for more muscular people). If you work out daily for 30 minutes over the course of a month, you will lose approximately 3600 calories; this is approximately equal to a pound of fat calories. After all this exercise you will only lose a pound! You can see how that can be frustrating.

The actual benefit of the exercise doesn't come from the calories spent during these thirty minutes. The actual benefit of the exercise is the boost to your metabolism. I will elaborate more about exercise and its benefit in a later chapter.

I want you to have realistic expectations and perspectives about why we do what we do to achieve weight loss. Exercise is one thing we do to improve our metabolism and our stamina, maintain lost weight, and it makes us happier while we are trying to lose weight.

You must drink water regularly to quench your thirst and keep hydrated; this will automatically work to cleanse and detox you

I have seen in many websites, journals, and in the media that if you need to detox that you must do certain things.

Do not fall into the trap of the mysterious detox procedures and spend money on it. It is very attractive; when you aren't happy with how you look or how you feel, to expect some magic wand that can "transform me."

Even I feel it sometimes. When we're busy with stress and not able to take care of ourselves, or when we feel sluggish and not like ourselves, we want to run out of our own selves and transform into something new.

Trust me, I get those feelings too.

One day, I went to get a haircut. It was at the end of a long working day, so I was tired. As I sat on the chair, I felt asleep.

My hairdresser knew me well; she waited until I woke up and then offered me juice to detox the fatigue while she did my hair.

I took the drink, as a detox sounded good, and because I love my hairdresser and her caring attitude.

On my way home, my stomach made a lot of noise; the minute I hit home I had a series of loose bowels.

It was because of this event that I looked into popular ways of detoxing our bodies.

Some so-called detox juices are made up of ingredients intended to stir up our gut: something acidic (sour), something spicy (pepper), and some stomach stimulants (concentrated sugar) to run your bowels. The purpose is to make it so you have a lot of bowel movements (frequent loose stools).

Basically, detox is a bowel stimulant; in other words, it's a glorified laxative.

But I admit, even I fell for it, because it sounded good. When you're tired, blah, and fatigued, you always hope for something to rescue you.

When you have several bowel movements due to intense stimulation of the bowel, you actually lose the gut's digestive juices along with electrolytes and lots of water (maybe few pounds of weight too, but this is not desirable as all you lose is water weight).

Weight loss this way is very unhealthy and dangerous. You run into dehydration, electrolyte imbalances (especially potassium and chloride), and even heart irregularities. Electrolyte balance is important for the heart to function correctly. As you can see, the ingredients in the juices are not bad, but the effects on the bowel's stimulation and the resulting electrolyte abnormalities can be detrimental. I have seen people admitted to the intensive care unit due to severe electrolyte abnormalities. Even though you may lose few pounds during a prolonged detoxing, what is lost is mainly water, not fat. If you are dehydrated, you cannot lose or burn fat at all. In fact when you are losing weight you are supposed to drink more water to burn fat.

By having frequent bowel movements, you don't remove the toxin from the body; instead the electrolytes and water are drawn out.

We don't accumulate toxins in our body, as one would think. A healthy liver will detox the body and the best way to keep the liver healthy is keeping it unburdened, primarily by keeping it free from unhealthy food.

The body experiences an oxidative stress that causes us to age as well as causes inflammation, fat accumulation, cellular degeneration, and cancers. Anti-oxidant effects and ways to reverse these toxic effects are discussed in a previous chapter.

Unfortunately, these detox techniques have no effect on improving or reversing the oxidative damage to our body.

💡 FAT-ME-NOT TIPS

SO HOW DO YOU DETOX YOUR BODY?

1. Drink 8 glasses of water daily.

2. Choose non-GMO meat and seafood.

3. Avoid artificial flavoring and sweeteners.

4. Limit sugar intake by choosing healthier snacks like nuts and fruit, and be sure to portion them correctly.

5. Get adequate amounts of sleep and rest.

WATER VS. SODA

This is my favorite discussion. We should drink water. **Just plain simple water**. Not flavored water. Not vitamin infused water. It doesn't matter if you're on a weight loss plan or not.

Drink an 8 ounce glass of water when you eat, when you feel thirsty, when you sweat, when you wake up, when you exercise, when you return from work/school, when you go to work/outside, and when you go to bed (assuming you don't have a frequent night time urination problem).

You should drink 8 glasses of water a day unless restricted by a physician. Just choose your time. The water gives you benefits such as those described below.

1. Energy

2. Freshness

3. Flushes out waste products

4. Regulates bowel movements

5. Keeps you in neutral taste

6. Cleans the mouth and oral cavity

7. Satisfies the stomach

8. Essential for a good weight-loss program

Too many medications may prevent you from losing weight

Evaluate all your medications with your doctor and categorize them as:

1. Must take medication
2. As-needed medication
3. Over-the-counter supplements

Review the side effects of weight gain with your doctor and ask if there are any possible alternatives.

Here are some medications that can cause weight gain, for which you may use some alternatives.

1. Steroids (prednisone)

    Alternatively, use these more selectively or use nasal sprays, topical creams, or joint injections rather than the pill or intravenous formulation.

2. Oral contraceptives

    Alternatively, use barrier methods or low hormone formulations. Don't use it just to regulate your period or just as a back up.

3. Psychotropics – medicines used to treat psychosis.

    a) Zyprexa (olanzapine)

    b) Lithium

    c) Clozaril (clozapine)

    d) Remeron (mirtazapine)

    e) Seroquel (quetiapine)

    f) Depakote (divalproex)

    g) Paxil (paroxetine)

h) Tricyclics (notriptyline, imipramine, doxepin)

Alternative weight-neutral antidepressants:

a) Lexapro (escitalopram)

b) Zoloft (sertraline)

c) Prozac (fluoxetine)

d) Wellbutrin (bupropion)

Alternative weight-neutral antipsychotics:

a) Aripiprazole (abilify)

b) Asenapine (saphrys)

c) Lurasidone (latuda)

d) Ziprasidone (geodon)

4. Insulin

Weight-neutral choices:

a) Lantus

b) Levemir

5. Thiazolinediones (actos, avandia)

Alternatively, use metformin

6. Sulfonylureas (glucotrol, glyburide, glimepiride)

Alternatively, use metformin (glucophage)

7. Beta blockers for hypertension or heart disease

For hypertension:

a) Metoprolol (lopressor)

b) Atenolol (tenormin)

Alternatively use weight-neutral beta-blocker: carvedilol (coreg)

8. Antiepileptics

a) Gabapentin

b) Pregabalin

c) Valproic acid

d) Carbamezapin

e) Vigabatrin

Alternative weight-neutral antiepileptics

a) Amotrigine

b) Levetiracetam

c) Phenytoin

Alternative weight-loss antiepileptics

a) Topiramate

b) Zonisamide

Give up artificial and natural sweeteners

So are there any non-alcoholic drinks that are intoxicating to the body?

We are seeing more and more evidence that drinking "diet drinks" regularly and in excess can harm your health. It is not healthy to drink, regardless of whether you are trying to lose weight or not.

I do clinically see in my practice that diet soda, in both regular and excess drinking, has caused migraines, headaches, foggy brain, lack of energy, fatigue, palpitations, mouth ulcers, and soreness. The literature has shown even more serious conditions caused by artificial sweeteners.

Sugary drinks include regular sodas, sports drinks, and sugar-added fruit juice; anything containing sugar can provide excessive calorie intake and increase your weight over time.

Approximately 500 excess calories per day can add a pound of fat per week.

Have you ever looked at the total calories per serving in what you drink? One 16 ounce bottle of soda contains 200 calories. Let's say you drink one bottle a day; you're guaranteed to gain one pound of fat in 2.5 weeks (seventeen days): approximately twenty pounds over a year.

Look at how many calories are in your drinks
1. When you're trying to maintain and/or lose weight, excessively or regularly drinking diet and non-diet soft drinks can give you extra calories, making you gain weight.
2. The diet soda calories don't satisfy you; instead, you crave more sugar.
3. You end up eating more than you would normally eat. (*Research has shown that people consume up to 40% more calories when they eat after consuming a diet drink.)

So do I give up on sodas and sugary drinks completely?

I personally do not drink diet drinks. When I drink, I drink regular drinks. They taste a lot better than diet ones anyways.

I pour out the soda into an ice-filled 8 ounce glass. I drink this 2-3 times a week, maximum. I have something else to snack on, like wholegrain crackers, nuts, cheese, or even potato chips. In brief, I drink soft drinks as a special drink snack. That is how the SlimPlate System's cold drink cup is designed too.

Yes, you will gain about 75 calories from the drink and another 75 calories from this snacking. However, when you mix simple sugars with complex sugars, protein, or fat, it prevents drastic ups and downs of sugar in the bloodstream and keeps your sugar levels steady. So it does not make you fatigued; you also don't crave more junk food to keep up your energy, so you end up eating less calories.

But I don't usually quench my thirst with soda, juice, or sport drinks. My regular daily drink is just plain water.

💡 FAT-ME-NOT TIPS

ROAD MAP TO TURNING OFF THE FAT SWITCH: STEPS YOU NEED DO TO TURN OFF THE FAT SWITCH

1. Drink eight glasses of water a day.
2. Eat breakfast regularly.
3. Eat regularly, including breakfast, lunch, dinner, and 1-2 snacks.
4. Eat regular food, not artificial foods like sweeteners.
5. Eat controlled portions as seen in the SlimPlate system.
6. Limit sugary drinks as this is the most common cause of fat accumulation in the body.
7. Do as much additional physical activity as you can daily that makes you sweat.

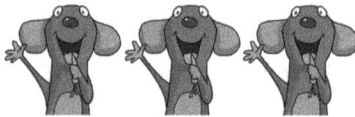

Fat-Me-Not success strategy

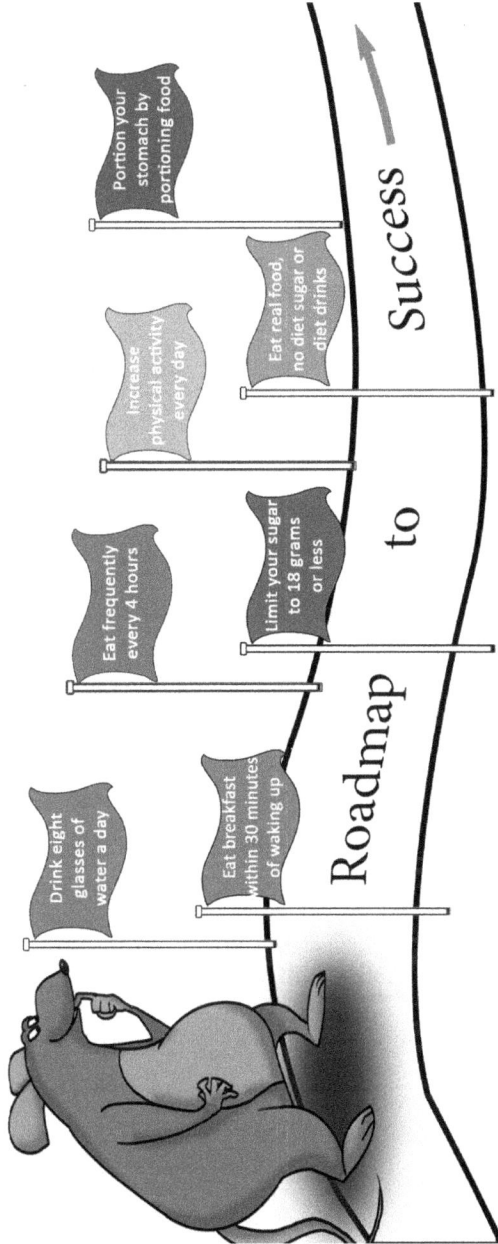

Chapter 5
Extraordinary Stories of Ordinary People

Learning From Their Experience

1. *The reasons I'm so committed to this mission: Loss of lives*

2. *Reunited: Woman fighting to save her marriage*

3. *Becoming a mother: Caring infertility*

4. *Self Esteem: A party girl achieves purpose*

5. *Because you care: On being a grandfather*

6. *A life changed: I can dance, I can jump, I can fly*

7. *Finally free: Ending a life of pain*

8. *A Caregiver: On taking care of herself*

9. *The three evils: Stress, Starvation, and Sugar*

The reasons I'm so committed to this mission: Loss of lives

I have done CPR and resuscitated many patients throughout my career. In this line of duty, we stay focused and within precise protocols; life and death is determined within the space of a few minutes. You might end up pronouncing a person dead, or, if the patient is lucky, they'll survive and be moved to an intensive care unit, given a second chance to live.

It's intense; you get less than ten minutes.

I have lost some of my patients. Even knowing that human beings are mortal, after every death I think about how we could have avoided it, if we could have achieved a different outcome.

The majority of obese people who don't survive resuscitation attempts suffer from either blood clots in the lungs or massive heart attacks. These two conditions are particularly common in young, obese patients.

I have lost three women and one man under the age of forty-five to a blood clot in the lung. The only disease they had in common was obesity. If they hadn't been obese, they might still be alive now, enjoying life on the young side of fifty.

Obesity kills. It kills quickly and there's nothing doctors can do to help patients at the edge of life and death. Even resuscitation is less effective in obese individuals. I always felt frightened, shocked, and helpless when trying to resuscitate very obese patients; that feeling never leaves me.

This is the reason I shout at the top of my voice that obesity kills. Don't become a victim of it.

Many people have successfully changed their lives by losing weight.

Reunited: Woman fighting to save her marriage

Jackie was a 35-year-old, 325 pounds obese woman. Her environment was her home, the computer, and her special chair. She was tired, had no energy, and couldn't do anything except for minor house chores.

When I first saw her she was expressionless and not interested in anything. She told me she was trying to save her marriage, and that she'd made the appointment to see me as a last ditch attempt to do so.

We bonded in our first meeting. I listened carefully to her difficulty in being active and her lack of motivation and energy; she didn't care if she got up or not the next day. She said she knew it wasn't right, but that was what she felt, and as a result she was in danger of losing her husband and her family.

In her case, obesity wiped out all of her energy and motivation and plunged her into depression. It had yet to kill her, but as a result of her obesity she lost many abilities enjoyed by 35-year-old women of normal weight.

We analyzed her problem through lab tests, her medical history, and an examination. Except for the fact that she was morbidly obese (a BMI of 40 or greater), her labs were normal. We assessed her dietary habit and discovered she lived on sugary drinks, a total of five 2-liter bottles per day, with only one meal at dinner.

Despite the fact that many patients suffering from obesity feel terrible, just as Jackie did, the majority of their labs return **normal**. Some return vitamin deficiencies such as D or B12, but this is usually the extent of their problems outside of obesity. Though we might expect that they would have additional problems, such as hormonal imbalances or renal and liver dysfunctions, but this is typically not the case.

I know that the reason my patients feel bad is because fat cells secrete inflammatory chemicals, making them feel sick. Basically, it's the fat itself that makes people feel bad all the time.

When patients begin to lose weight, they start feeling better. Once the sickening effects of the chemicals secreted by fat tissue are stunted and begin to recede, patients begin to experience improved health and feeling of well-being. I've observed this in many of my patients, and refer to it as their turning point.

Once we saw the problems in her dietary habits, the solution wasn't that difficult to find. We put her on the Fat-Me-Not success plan (this will be discussed in greater detail in a later chapter). We worked with her to break the habit of constantly consuming sugary drinks, breaking the constant fat-saving mode in the process.

By the end of the first month, Jackie had lost 23 pounds. I can still hear her shrieking with excitement; the expressionless woman turned into a young woman enthused about life. At that point, she became more convinced that she could successfully lose weight. She understood how, by eating frequently and not exceeding her daily sugar limit, she could enjoy many kinds of food and still lose weight biologically.

After five months, the two of us had a little victory dance in the clinic room. She said that the treatment helped her save her marriage. With obesity now a thing of the past, Jackie is able to look forward, convinced that she'd now be able to be a young, healthy, and happily married woman.

At present, Jackie weighs 207 pounds and is the proud owner of a successful home interior decorating company.

Becoming a mother: Curing infertility

Teresa was a 33-year-old, happy southern girl who married her high school sweetheart. She worked in a kindergarten, but though she played with babies and toddlers every day at work, she and her husband had been unsuccessful at having a child of their own. Her gynecologist referred her to our weight loss clinic, which is how she ended up coming to see me.

Despite having been married for twelve years, Theresa had never gotten pregnant. She became very emotional when talking about her history of weight gain, and it became very obvious that she had no idea that her inability to get pregnant was because of her excess weight. She felt guilty and blamed herself for failing to get pregnant as she confided in me her past attempts to lose weight.

Since her early 20s, Theresa had tried a number of the diet plans on the market, with disappointing results: she ended up gaining 80 pounds rather than losing any weight at all.

We scratched all of that and started her on the Fat-Me-Not success plan. Using the SlimPlate System portion plates and cups, Theresa continued eating her own home cooked southern food. She followed the success strategy thoroughly and gave up her habit of drinking diet soda. As a result, she is now in charge of her weight rather than her weight dominating her.

I worked with Theresa for over an hour with the Fat-Me-Not success plan, as I do with everyone who comes through our program. Like everyone else who leaves our program, Theresa left feeling reassured and contented with the road ahead. She went home with the success plan drawn out in detail, a portion control set, and a sense of satisfaction

As I expected, she lost weight and was able to conceive a beautiful baby.

On a bright, sunny day, Theresa came and showed us her beautiful baby boy. Every morning, she pulls on a size 10 outfit and goes out to push her baby stroller; her old size 22 clothes have been retired to the back of her closet.

Losing weight can change your life. I always say that weight loss is fun: you're in charge of who you can become.

Self Esteem: A party girl achieves purpose

Yvonne was an 18-year-old girl; she came to see me for her physical. A few days later, her Pap smear came back positive for a high-risk strain of Human Papilloma Virus (HPV).

HPV can increase the risk of cervical cancer in young women, so I called Yvonne back in to discuss her options.

As I went through the risks of HPV and how it was transmitted, I noticed that Yvonne didn't seem particularly worried, despite her youth. I wanted to make sure she understood the information I was giving her, so in an effort to learn more about her I started to chat with her more casually; I found out that she was a college student, studying art. She gradually opened up to me and admitted that she'd had a startling number of sexual partners.

I quickly discovered that Yvonne's toughness was only on the surface. She was incredibly ashamed of her weight, to the point that she thought that no one would ever want to be with her. It was for this reason that she had had numerous sexual partners already — she was willing to let anyone use her body in order to feel wanted.

This made me incredibly sad; I hugged her for a long time before she left that day. I told her to come back, that we were going to tackle this problem and change it.

Yvonne is six feet tall; when she first came to me, she weighed about 278 pounds.

I put her on the Fat-Me-Not success plan and had her stay on the SlimPlate portion control plates. She also started playing tennis. Instead of trying a get a quick fix, Yvonne followed the plan; with every step she completed, she solidified her success. She wrote down the Fat-Me-Not Success Strategy and placed it in the small frame on her study table so that she'd be reminded of the plan every day. She didn't use any kind of medication to lose weight.

Yvonne lost 85 pounds in 10 months and with her newfound confidence, she's started a career as a performer in a regional theater.

Don't ignore how important feeling great about yourself every day is to achieving a healthy weight. It's a powerful feeling, and keeping hold of it can help you attain your goals; without that positivity, you can easily find yourself dragged down into despair.

Because you care: On being grandfather

We live in a society where we care about each other. Parents care about their kids; children care about their parents, especially as they grow older. Husbands care about their wives; wives care about their husbands. Grandchildren, friends, and families care about each other. Even in our work environments, we care about the people we work with; it's important to each of us that others care for us, and we take pride in caring for others.

It's important to be able to stay in this circle of care.

I know a man who goes by Grandpa Paul; he received a gift from his son, to see me at my weight loss clinic, and came in with a two-year-old boy.

Grandpa Paul was in his early sixties and weighed 387 pounds. He was babysitting his grandson on the day he came to see me. We were in a big conference room, Grandpa Paul, the little boy, playing on the floor and me. He often had to reach down to pick up his grandson; this caused him difficulty, and for several minutes after picking up the little boy he was unable to catch his breath.

During the course of conversation, I learned that Grandpa Paul was a plumber; no longer able to perform his work, he had started staying home with his son's family to take care of his grandson. He said to me, "Hit me, doc. I got nothing to do at home. I'm all yours and ready to lose some weight so I can play with this little fellow again."

I was convinced and told him that with that kind of motivation he'd be playing with his grandson again in a month. The most important thing for Grandpa Paul was that he wanted to play with the little boy again; his smile told me that he was already imagining that eventuality.

The obesity hadn't taken his life, but it had severely reduced his mobility and made his breathing difficult.

We laid out the Fat-Me-Not success plan; he was drinking way too many sweet drinks. Grandpa Paul cut out the success plan and put it in his wallet as a constant reminder.

I saw him again after six weeks instead of the usual four, and at that point he'd lost 28 pounds and was able to play with his grandson again. Now, he's been on the weight loss program for seven months and is down to 285 pounds. I haven't seen his grandson again, but Grandpa Paul is back in uniform, working for a plumbing company on a city project.

He's now able to bend down and take off his work boots. The last time he came to see me, he told me that he'd been looking forward to the weigh-in all month. Since he's begun losing weight, playing with his grandson has been a lot more fun.

Grandpa Paul came to see me because he is part of a circle of care. It's important that we pause and think sometimes; what makes us healthy makes the people around us feel happy, and then we feel happy in turn.

For me, the health of my family, friends, and patients is the most important thing in my life. Helping these people maintain their health gives me personal satisfaction.

A life changed: I can dance, I can jump, I can fly

Susan came to see me in my primary care clinic for years due to knee joint pain that kept getting worse. We did a bilateral knee x-ray, and after looking at the scans I told her how we were going to fix the problem.

I said I'd give her medication for pain relief, but her joints were inflamed from the bones scraping against each other as she walked. The pain medications were only a temporary fix; without addressing the problem more directly, she'd end up taking the pain meds for the rest of her life, and would have to deal with side effects, including drowsiness.

Susan was only 42-years-old and she weighed about 265 pounds. Knee prostheses weren't an option, as they're reserved for older people; they need to be replaced approximately every ten years. The other problem with prostheses is that they are made for people at normal weights rather than individuals struggling with obesity. Often, the point of pain will shift to where the bone and prosthesis connect.

If Susan were to get a new knee, she'd end up having to repeat the surgery every ten years, even if the pain were resolved by the surgery. With pain in both knees, that would be two surgeries every ten years. With each surgery, there would be a recovery time of approximately six months.

Susan asked me what her future was likely to look like. I pulled out a post-it and drew a person with a cane, then labeled it as "Now". On a second post-it, I drew a person with a walker and labeled it as "Two Years". On a third post-it, I drew a person in a wheelchair and labeled it as "5 Years".

You can imagine how hard it would be for a 42-year-old lady to learn that she might be in a wheelchair by the age of 47, when she doesn't have any diseases other than obesity. It was terrible to have to tell someone I care that unless she took immediate steps, she would be confined to a wheelchair within five years. Admittedly, this prediction isn't 100% accurate, but even if it's only 50% accurate, it's a big risk to take.

Susan asked me what she needed to do to avoid the future I had laid out for her. As you probably figured out, I told her she needed to lose weight.

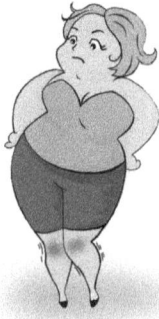
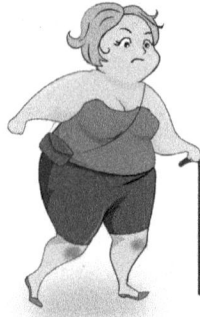

Now   In one year

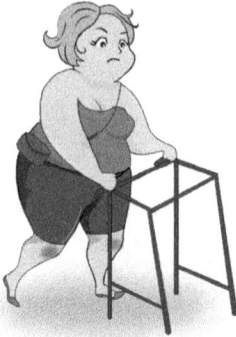
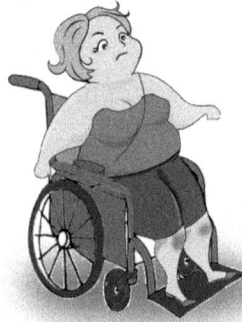

In 3 years   In 5 years

I treated her with NSAIDs anti-inflammatories and painkillers to relieve her pain and suggested that she try participating in water aerobics at the local YMCA. And, of course, I urged her to lose weight.

By losing weight, Susan gained two benefits. Reducing the fat mass (weight) reduced the grinding impact of bone against bone as well as the inflammation in the body. The less weight she carried, the better her joint inflammation got.

Susan was an otherwise healthy young woman; she just needed a wake up call. When she left the clinic, she took my post-it drawings with her. She started her weight loss journey at our Ace Medical Weight Loss Center, where we put her on the Fat-Me-Not success plan. Since starting the plan, she's dropped down to 197 pounds. The last time she came into the clinic, she was full of joy, and showed me a picture of my post-it drawings stuck to her nightstand, where she could see them every day. I practice both primary care and obesity medicine. Many of my patients have successfully completed my formal weight loss program, but some of them were unable to finish. Our formal weight loss program includes diet, exercise, lifestyle changes and behavioral improvement, and optional medication.

Most patients unable to go through with the formal program are elderly or disabled; often they can't come to the clinic easily due to transportation issues. Unfortunately, they're the people who need this service the most.

I made a special online weight-loss program for them, where they can listen from home at their convenience and learn how to use the Fat-Me-Not success plan. Many of my physically disabled patients have gone on the online weight-loss program and have lost weight, improving their health. You are welcome to join this program free at www.slimplatesystem.com. Just enter your email and you will receive instructions on where to access my weight loss teachings.

In my primary care practice (not weight loss clinic), I see my patients every three months; most put on weight with each successive visit. The way we currently eat in the United States means we consume way too many calories and consequently gain about 13-26 pounds every year. The only way to resist is systematic portion control. Many of my patients use the SlimPlate System; they are the proof that portion control helps with weight.

Many physically disabled patients are able to steadily lose weight. Though they're physically limited, they can't do a lot to spend additional calories, but they are able to learn to eat right to improve their metabolism, resulting in significant weight loss.

Imagine losing two pounds a month, on average, instead of gaining two pounds a month by eating right. At the end of the year, you'd be twenty-four pounds lighter than when you started, and forty-eight pounds lighter than if you'd not done anything to lose weight at all. This is the right way to go about controlling your weight: before you start a weight-loss program, you need to be sure it will result in sustained weight loss.

If you have any physical disabilities or are in a wheelchair, start using the easy, simple guide to success that the Fat-Me-Not Success plan offers — start eating right, with a balanced diet and follow all steps. Or you can also consider using SlimPlate System to make it easier.

Finally free: Ending a life of pain

Joy and John always come to see me in my medical practice. John is a sick man and a cancer survivor, but he's still a happy person. Even though he wears a tracheostomy — a hole in his windpipe — he always strikes to me as a happy person.

A person with a tracheostomy can do only one thing at a time; they can breathe, or in order to talk, they close off the hole, usually with a finger. He mostly stays quiet and smiles when he's with his wife.

But one day, John came to see me alone. He had been married to Joy for eight years and he was concerned because she hadn't been happy. As I listened to him, I realized that she often cried, became very apologetic at times, and constantly explained why she did what she did.

I asked John how and why this behavior bothered him.

John explained that he loved her, but didn't want to be near her because she was angry all the time and then cried. This was perfectly understandable.

I asked him what was bothering her.

He told me that she hurt all over.

With that, I figured out the answer.

Pain isn't easy, and it's unpleasant feeling that can bring you down.

I comforted John and promised that I would talk to Joy about how we could improve her pain.

Joy, who weighed 256 pounds and stood 63 inches tall, came back and saw me. I had spoken with her husband in private, but I was prepared to help her with her pain.

I'd already guessed what is her problem is. The most important part was to make Joy understand her problem.

I gave her a notepad with a picture of a person and asked her to mark where she felt discomfort or pain.

She marked her right hip, her back, her knees, her upper back, her feet... and then it became all over. Then she laughed and said, "I've marked my entire body, haven't I?"

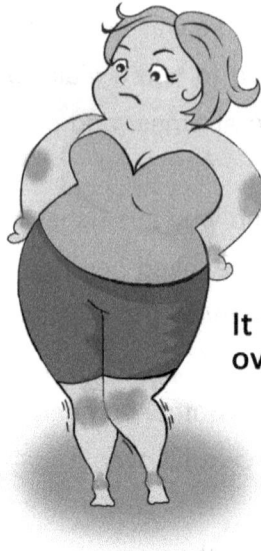

It hurts all over my body

She explained that she had bad arthritis throughout her body and that she hurt when she moved. She'd forgotten the last time she had a pain-free moment. She felt really bad about being angry, and crying, because she had money, a husband, great step-kids — it was just that she lived in pain.

Admitting this, she became emotional and started crying. She told me that she didn't want to get out of bed in the morning. She hated depending on someone else for help, but because of the pain she needed to wait for someone to help her do things. She explained that her husband was older, and sick, so she felt bad that she needed to depend on him to pull her out of bed and help her put on her shoes and socks. Because of the constant pain, she was always in a bad mood and would get angry and raise her voice if people didn't do things right or caused her pain, and as a result she would then feel sad and guilty. She explained that sometimes she'd try to do things herself, so she didn't have to bother anyone, but then felt even worse when she wasn't able to do it. All of this meant that she just felt hopeless on top of always feeling bad.

I choked up listening to her.

Then I asked her if she knew why her body hurt.

She answered that she had arthritis — inflammation of the joints. She said she was taking arthritis medications, but that didn't help.

I asked her if she hurt all over, not just at the joints, but also at her muscles, like at her shoulders. She nodded, so I asked her if she knew why her joints and muscles were inflamed, and then I explained that "sick fat syndrome" was responsible for her pain.

What is sick fat?

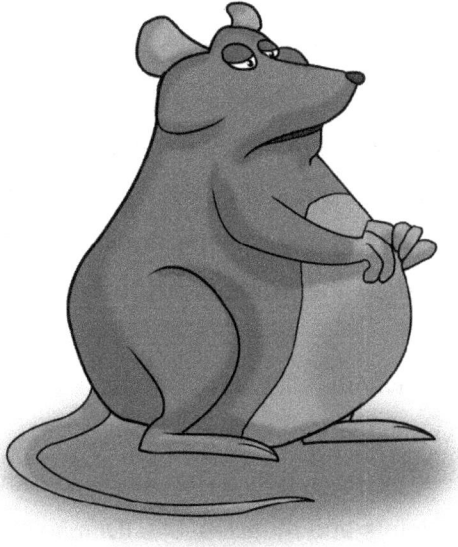

As we all know, too much of a good thing isn't good. The body needs fat, and fat does have many health benefits. But if we let too much fat accumulate, it reverses all the good things fat can do for the body. Basically, our bodies go into an "inflamed mode" and the body becomes sick. As a result, disaster strikes the body in the form of sick fat syndrome.

The sick fat creates an overwhelming inflammatory reaction in body that causes obesity-related sickness.

1. Inflammation
2. Tissue hypoxia (lack of Oxygen)
3. Neurodegeneration (memory loss, depression, lack of energy, degeneration of the nervous system)
4. Abnormal glucose metabolism (diabetes)
5. Atherosclerosis (hard or blocked arteries)
6. Endocrinopathy (hormone problems)
7. Multiple cancers

In our body, sick fat causes abnormal cell function, and triggers the degeneration process. This sick fat secretes chemicals, which starts a cascade of inflammation throughout the body. Essentially, the sick fat changes the state of our body, making it unhealthy.

Obesity doesn't just involve one organ. It's an overwhelming condition that affects the whole body and sickens the organs, including:

1. Fatty liver- where fat invades the liver
2. Poorly ventilated lung (Sleep apnea)
3. Decreased blood supply to heart. (Heart attacks)
4. Inflamed joints and muscles, etc. (Diffuse pain)
5. Chronic fatigue (Lack of energy)
6. Blood vessel diseases
7. Sick brain (stroke)

With sick fat syndrome, being morbidly obese or being one hundred pounds over ideal weight can cause the organs in your body to become sick. This includes women who weigh over 230 pounds and men who weigh over 250 pounds.

It's a depressing thing to realize, isn't it? But here's something to cheer you up: lose about 10% of your body weight — around 20-30 pounds, depending on your initial weight — and you'll find yourself transformed. Lose the weight, and all of your sick fat syndrome symptoms will vanish along with it. Your pain will improve; your energy will return; your breathing will be better; and on the whole, you'll look and feel better.

Losing weight is worth it. It can be fun, because by losing weight, all of the good things you thought you had lost will return to your life.

So I had a long discussion with Joy. I told her that we would work through her pain together and that we would come out the other side successfully. She positively sparkled with hope.

It wasn't false hope. It's the kind of results that everyone can achieve.

You might argue and point out that Joy couldn't even bend down to tie her shoe; how was she going to get on a treadmill or work out and lose weight?

When they first come to me, many of my patients aren't able to move more than few yards; medication isn't an option, either, due to comorbid heart diseases.

Our body's powerful metabolism actually helps us reset our weight control.

Someone who's been overwhelmed with sick fat syndrome has essentially lost his or her body's weight control mechanism.

Unfortunately, no magic pill can turn on the metabolism's power.

There is one way that you can turn your metabolism around. I have found this strategy through consultation with patients, as well as my knowledge on obesity. I named it the Fat-Me-Not success plan.

In my many years of practicing medicine, the Fat-Me-Not success plan is the simplest strategy that I've found, one that everyone can accomplish easily and successfully. The Fat-Me-Not plan will be discussed in a later chapter.

I laid out the success play for Joy and explained that she had to give up drinking diet soda, re-learn drinking water, and eat breakfast regularly. She followed these rules and saw changes in her energy levels, as well as changes in her food behaviors.

Joy told me that since starting the Fat-Me-Not success plan, she'd started to look forward to eating breakfast when she woke up in the morning. All these little changes told me that she was resetting her metabolism. She actually started feeling hungry at mealtimes and lost the constant desire to drink diet soda. Before starting the plan, she felt like she could go all day without eating anything, surviving only on diet drinks.

She followed the plan. Three months into it, I noticed she was able to complete a visit to the clinic without breaking down in tears. She acted like an enthusiastic little girl, eagerly looking forward to each forthcoming moment.

Do you know what all these little changes mean?

The overwhelming inflammation in her body was receding, losing the attempt to take over her body and her metabolism.

Joy was able to defeat her body's inflammation. By the ninth month on the plan, she weighed forty-six pounds lighter than she had when she started.

As a result, she wasn't in constant pain and she no longer cried at the drop of a hat. I could see her bright and infectious smile from far away.

Best of all, she was in charge of her body and once again independent.

With this in mind, tell me why would you want to stay in pain? Why would you want to ignore the fact that you can get rid of the pain?

A Caregiver: On taking care of herself

Julie is the mother of a disabled adult son. The son was born with cerebral palsy, a type of congenital brain injury that required multiple surgeries; multiple seizures left him paralyzed and non-communicative.

This, as you might imagine, was a major stress in her life. Julie single-handedly took care of her son.

Julie came to me and told me that her son had another bladder infection.

I asked her how she knew, as her son was non-communicative. What I really wanted to know was what symptoms her son had that made her think he had a bladder infection.

She told me that in the previous fourteen hours he'd been kicking harder and harder and that his face had been getting pinker. She described how, in the space of an hour, he'd grimaced fifteen times, and explained that for thirty-six hours his urine had been cloudy, and that he was drawing closer to the left side of his groin.

These were the details she knew about her son. Her son wasn't able to communicate and wasn't aware of his surroundings; as a result of his brain injury, he didn't get fevers in the same way as others.

Julie moved her son, transferring him from his chair to his bed, or to other places; she took him to the park, on road trips, and shopping. It was a big challenge to take care of a man as totally disabled as he was, by herself, but she did it anyways.

She constantly talked to him, explained things to him, and communicated with him as though he could understand her. She also learned his body language by observing every movement that he made.

Julie was morbidly obese and suffered from pain in several of her joints. Her back caused her severe pain and she had to take 5-8 goody powders a day. Every single time she came to see me, always with her son, she had put on more weight.

At that point, Julie wasn't my regular patient. She only came in once in a while when she wasn't able to tolerate her back pain. She kept her visits short; she just wanted to get pain medications, and she rarely talked about anything else that troubled her. She repeatedly postponed routine checkups like blood draws and mammograms, politely saying that she'd have it done at her next appointment.

One day, Julie went to the ER with crushing chest pain. When she came out of the hospital, it was with a mended heart and a large scar on her chest. Right after she came out of the hospital, her son went into the hospital with overwhelming infection (septic shock). He stayed in the hospital for weeks before returning to live with her.

That was a wakeup call for Julie.

Sometime after that, she came to see me and asked me to do complete physical exam and run all of the tests that I'd wanted to do but she previously kept putting it off. After a few visits, I had diagnosed her as diabetic, with heart disease, bad cholesterol, severe disc disease in her back, severely arthritic knees, fatty liver, and severe sleep apnea.

She had every problem that can be caused by obesity.

If you aren't obese, you may get one or two of these conditions, but it's unlikely you'll get all of them in rapid succession.

Similar heart diseases happen in non-obese patients, but these patients are unlikely to also have sleep apnea, fatty liver and back pain all at the same time.

That is what I explain to my patients as an obesity syndrome. It affects every part of the body simultaneously and in various ways.

When you suffer from obesity syndrome, finding shelter can be very hard. This is what frightens me the most.

- An overwhelming amount of fat growth in the body makes us feel incredibly sick. It causes inflammation in the body.
- It thickens our blood and can cause blood clots.
- It thickens our arteries and can cause blockages. It deprives our tissue of oxygen.
- It releases various toxins.
- It alters bodily functions, including breathing, digestion, circulation, and reproduction.
- It destroys our normal metabolism and control systems.
- It destroys our nervous system and causes constant fatigue.
- It can cause abnormal cell and tissue growth and cause cancers.

How can we reverse this process? We cannot stop it by:

- Not eating
- Limiting food
- Wiring the jaw
- Patching the tongue
- Going on a low-calorie diet
- Taking 'magic' pills, powders, or oils

None of these tactics will work because unfortunately, there aren't any fat-dissolving tools that will simply remove fat from the body. This has to come from within. Your metabolism has to work to digest and utilize its fat. Only then can the sick fat leave the body.

We are human and we are biological. This is why something that sounds logical just won't work. Shakes, pills, and lotion — these won't help you lose the fat inside your body.

We can't fool the brain for long; it will find out. Later in this book we'll discuss abnormal eating behaviors.

The best way to stop is to give your body a chance to return to normal by:

- Consuming a balanced diet
- Allowing your body to function normally
- Eat real food and let your digestive system do its job normally
- Get sufficient hydration
- Allow for the natural thermogenic effect of food
- Eliminate abnormal eating behaviors by eating regular food in a balanced diet

Julie was in shock when she found out about all of her conditions; it was entirely unreal to her.

Unfortunately, I wasn't surprised that she suffered from so many problems. She'd weighed around 345 pounds for many years and she'd ignored her weight, not seeing it as a problem.

Increased body weight is an abnormality, not a vanity issue. It really affects your health.

Ask yourself a few simple questions: What is my normal weight? What is my current weight?

I suggest the following limits, based on a complicated scientific calculation.

A six-foot tall woman shouldn't weigh more than 180 pounds.

A five-foot tall woman shouldn't weigh more than 120 pounds.

A six-foot tall man shouldn't weigh more than 200 pounds.

A five-foot tall man shouldn't weigh more than 135 pounds.

I've had patients tell me to give them a break — that they haven't weighed less than 180 pounds since they were eighteen. The truth is, if that's the case then you've been overweight since childhood.

I've also heard patients say that back then, they were healthy; nothing hurt them. They slept well, their cholesterol was good, and they didn't have any trouble with diabetes. Now, at 250 pounds, they have all of these problems.

Our body organs come with regenerating power and the ability to adapt. For example, if you lose one kidney, the other kidney will take over and compensate for the loss, and you still can live your full life span. If you lose lung function due to smoking, your body can compensate so that you can breathe normally long-term, and then for a longer lifespan oxygen supplementation can help. With obesity, the body can regenerate, repair and compensate until the percentage of fat in the body becomes an overwhelming problem.

Over the course of three months, we got Julie's diabetes, pain, and cholesterol under control; to do just this, she went from taking zero medications to taking twelve pills. This was just to get her immediate problems under control; the medication couldn't cure them, because without effective weight-loss, these conditions can't be cured.

Julie still has to take all of these medications to keep her conditions under control, but unfortunately she also suffers the many side effects of the drugs, including drowsiness.

Here, I'd like to point out a few things about medications.

As a doctor, I know that medications come with side effects.

But the bigger evils are heart attacks, back pain, diabetes…the list goes on and on. If these conditions are out of control, your life is in danger. For instance, complications with uncontrolled diabetes can very quickly become destructive to the body.

So we have to choose the lesser evil. Taking medications, and dealing with their side effects, means that we can deal with the bigger evils of high sugar and high cholesterol, etc.

My patients often also want to know what they can do to combat their conditions naturally, without having to go on any kind of medication.

'Natural' is a powerful word. We hear about natural substances, natural ways — people think that "natural" means "safe", and so they go and buy things that are labeled natural. Multi-billion dollar industries are built on products advertised as being "natural" in some way, because people desperately want to believe in natural hormones, natural ways to lose cholesterol, natural ways to control diabetes…

Without going into further details, I will remind you of one thing:

Tornadoes, earthquakes, tsunamis, and storms are all natural, not manmade. More specifically, they are natural disasters. "Natural" doesn't always equate to "better" or "safer".

Medications go through multiple large-scale studies. Studies must first be done on animals, then on healthy humans, and then specific diseased humans. Finally specific efficacy and safety studies are done. It is a long, tedious, and expensive process to get medications approved for sale on the market.

Every single medication has side effects, but these are observed, tracked, and known as a result of the studies, and are listed on every medication. When you know the side effects of a medication, you are able to weigh them against the benefit.

Over-the-counter medication, however, rarely go through any controlled studies. No side effects are listed, as they are not tracked and therefore are not known; this doesn't mean that there aren't dangerous side effects.

Natural substances can still have many side effects, but they are not listed on the packaging, nor are they systematically compiled or studied. Their efficacy is not quantified, their side effects are not tracked and followed, and their proper uses are not observed and studied.

We use these supplements with very little knowledge, and as a result we're walking on thin ice.

I've seen many patients consume different over–the-counter, natural supplements, and many of them have suffered as the supplements do not have enough efficacy or they are incompatible with the human body.

For example, there is a lot of information about garlic helping to lower cholesterol. Garlic is not dangerous to take, but on its own it isn't enough to lower cholesterol to a healthy level. On top of that, we don't know how much a pill, or a clove of garlic, per day lowers cholesterol.

This is why dismissing medications in favor of natural supplements really isn't the way to go. If you have something like high cholesterol, it's a good idea to include garlic in your diet, but you also need to take the appropriate medications to keep your cholesterol in check so that you don't suffer from stroke or heart attack later on.

That being said, I'm a big advocate of not taking medication if it is not needed, so in a way I'm a naturalist too. I hate medications — for me the best thing is that we all are healthy and no one needs to take any medications at all.

This is the first and foremost reason I became an obesity specialist: to prevent disease before it has a chance to take root, and to help eradicate disease when it's already present.

Let's continue with Julie. We'd just stabilized for her medical conditions with twelve different medications. She faithfully took her medications, even though she didn't like to. As a result of shortness of breath and almost unbearable back pain, she had limited mobility; she'd begun to realize that she was going to have a problem, going forward trying to continue taking care of her adult, disabled son.

We went through a series of investigations on her back and tried back injections for back pain, which resulted in temporary fixes. A neurosurgical evaluation told us that she wasn't a candidate for invasive surgery as she has moderately severe pulmonary hypertension due to her sleep apnea.

Sometimes in medical practice, doctors do get stuck like this.

Julie joined a famous commercial weight-loss program right after her heart surgery. She initially lost a few pounds, but in time she saw that she was getting worse. Finally, when she reached 402 pounds, she asked for my help.

I embarked on her weight-loss journey to help her. First and foremost, I told her that this was a lifestyle change; the habits we started her on would last forever. I don't have magic, but I do know how to improve the metabolism.

Julie and I planned how to fight fat based on her food choices and what her day looked like.

When my patients are working on losing weight, I don't want them to think that they have to move mountains. We can't move mountains forever. We can't be constantly running marathons. Julie was a far cry from running marathons; she could barely walk to her car.

We can't stay on celery sticks and chicken breasts forever. It isn't right to eat non-nutrient vegetables like celery and salad to lose weight. I don't recommend my patients to eat salad at all. I personally don't like salad and almost never eat them.

I taught Julie to focus on what she could do that was compatible with her lifestyle, and told her to do it repeatedly.

She was put on a plan that focused on the right amount of real food at the right times, with instructions to repeat that day after day. With that formula, she used her SlimPlate system very regularly.

Julie started to shed weight. I coached her monthly, though in the beginning it was hard because of all her comorbid conditions.

One thing I've noticed is that once they shed about 5% of their body weight, people start feeling better. In Julie's case, she lost 21 pounds in the first few months, was subsequently in less pain and was less tense throughout her body.

This is what stunts the pro-inflammatory state. The sick fat swells and inflames the body, making us feel sluggish, draggy, and fatigued, as well as constantly in pain. Once it is reduced, symptoms start getting better.

I explained to Julie at every step what the process was achieving, beyond just losing the weight. She became more and more motivated. She grew happier. It was like she started seeing her own life. She had been living only for her son's, and had never known how to live for herself.

She slowly became choosier in her daily life, eating more creatively. She'd spent many years eating quick-fix macaroni and cheese, but now she started to enjoy different foods. She never used to pay attention to fixing good things for herself to eat, or be interested in trying different recipes, because her son is fed by a tube. Now, however, she takes an interest in what she eats and takes her vitamins regularly.

She saw the light at the end of the tunnel, where she could be if she lost the weight. This is what I want my patients to achieve. I want them to realize that they are in charge of their lives. Life is full of surprises; we don't know what's ahead of us —we just have to be curious to what comes next.

Once you are curious about life, you'll be able to achieve your goals.

Julie has dropped down to 300 pounds. She hadn't dated a man in twenty years, but now she's got a sweet gentleman as a walking partner.

She might not have reached her goal yet, but she's gained confidence to live on and the ability to live a new life.

The three evils: Stress, Starvation, and Sugar

Brenda, who suffers from bipolar disorder and sees a psychiatrist, came to see me in the clinic one day. This wasn't a usual experience, so I still remember it.

She had come for a follow-up. I checked her vitals. Her vitals were fine, but her blood pressure was up a little and she'd gained a few pounds. I asked her if anything had changed in the previous there months; she shook her head.

I asked her if she'd eaten anything that morning, so we could check her labs.

We went over her medications and I asked her if there had been any changes. She told me some of her psychiatric medications had been increased. I was thinking; she was quiet and tense. Then I noticed her face was red.

Then I rolled my chair closer to her and asked softly if anything was bothering her.

She suddenly jumped out of her chair and stood against the wall furthest from me. Her words came out in out bursts.

"You are the same as everyone else, nothing different. My parents like you; they think the world of you. Church people said you walk on water. So I came to see you. But you're just like others. You don't understand me. You don't know me. You all just come up with all these accusations."

As you might imagine, I was shocked. I felt like someone had thrown water on my face, which was red and hot.

I ran back over the situation in my head, trying to figure out what I'd done to make her mad, but couldn't think of anything.

So what had upset her?

Then she started crying, tears rolling down her cheeks.

The silence went on. She had a few more outbursts, said a few more offensive things. After some initial heat, I was able to control myself, and I looked at her carefully. She was like a threatened kitten, frightened and ready to attack and fight back. All her claws were out and she was ready to jump, but at the same time, she couldn't stop crying.

All of a sudden, I realized that something was about to happen.

My daily schedule is busy. Usually patients are scheduled every fifteen minutes at the clinic, and I'm usually booked up continuously from nine in the morning until four in the afternoon. Except for a quick lunch, I don't get a break. I'm always aware that patients will be waiting for me in the other five exam rooms, so I make an effort to stay on time.

But this was an important moment, and I didn't want to miss it, even though the room was hot and I was stressed.

After a long silence, I observed that it was getting warm in the room. I said I want to get a glass of water and asked if she wanted one.

She said No.

I excused myself for few seconds and brought back two cups of water. I left the door ajar to cool down the room.

I left one cup of water next to her and then sat back down.

I took a few sips of water, and was ready to find out what was bothering her.

"I'm sorry that I said something to upset you," I told her. "I didn't mean to do so."

She took a half breath and said, "People don't know me. Even my doctor doesn't know me."

I smiled at her, acknowledging her words. I didn't want to interrupt; I wanted her to continue talking.

She told me that when I last saw her, I told her that she had gained 112 lbs over the previous year. Since then she hadn't eaten any food, but was angry because she'd gained thirty-seven pound since the last time she had seen me.

What she said was true. I noticed that she remembered the conversation from three months earlier, when she admitted that she knew she'd gained weight. I also remembered that visit. I was concerned about her weight gain, but when I mentioned it she didn't seem like she cared; she just interrupted me. Because of this, this time I hadn't specifically mentioned how much weight she'd gained since the last time I'd seen her; I didn't want to upset her. It turned out that she already knew she'd gained a lot of weight.

She cared how much she weighed, and she knew that she was gaining weight despite trying to lose weight by not eating.

At that point, I knew exactly what was going on with her. This is the thing about being a doctor: sometimes we catch things, little things that let us figure out what's going on with our patients. We're trained to pick out the important, relevant facts out from a lengthy conversation.

Brenda said she hadn't eaten any food since the last time she had seen me. That was about three months.

I believed that she was telling the truth.

She was in stress mode, a hyper-adrenaline state. Her face was red and super sensitive; she was in a fight-or-flight mode. This was exacerbated by not eating.

She wanted to know why she had gained thirty-seven pounds when she hadn't eaten anything in months.

She was still standing against the wall, still in super-sensitive mode.

I told her to come over and sit down, that we'd talk about it.

She reluctantly came and sat down.

I gave her the water. She took it this time and took few sips.

I repeated that she hadn't been eating, and then asked if she was ever hungry. She said she had been, but not anymore. Then she began to cry again. She said she'd found out she had gained thirty-seven pounds despite not eating, and wanted to know how this was possible.

I gave her a few napkins and waited for her to wipe her tears. Then I picked up the flyer and fanned her to help cool her down.

I almost knew already how she had survived during three months without eating. I guess that comes from many similar conversations with my patients.

During the three months, she drank Mountain Dew to relieve her hunger — between three and five two-liter bottles per day, every day, during the previous three months.

Stress, Starvation and Sugar. I could clearly see that these three had thoroughly destroyed her body, putting it into a bad shape. This is the worst combination for damaging the body.

I got my answer. I was satisfied. I knew how to fix this.

I touched her hand gently in reassurance.

I wrote down a few lab tests, including some to check hormone levels (thyroid, stress hormones, female hormones, insulin, and chemistry).

I told her to get the blood tests done and then to come and see me the next day, thirty minutes earlier than the clinic start time. Then I said, smiling, that tomorrow we'd walk on water.

She smiled back at me, her eyes twinkling; I knew she believed what I'd said.

As I came out of the room, I was embraced by my super-efficient nurses, who told me about all the rooms that were waiting for me and what had been done, and I put my imaginary skate wheel on.

But I was wearing a big smile. I was happy; I knew how to fix Brenda's problem.

Stress, Starvation, and Sugar

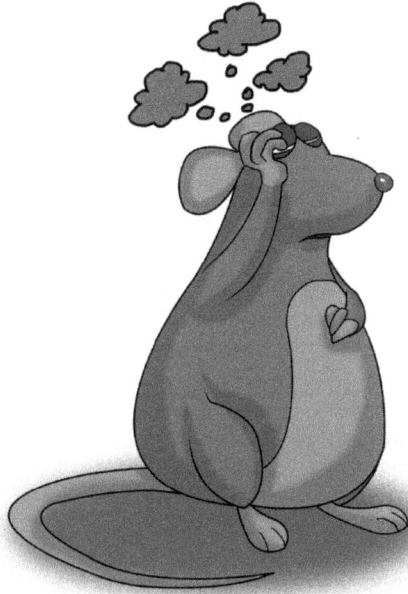

STRESS

Stress causes the body to swell and puts us into a disorganized mode.

1. Excessive glucose production causes diabetes
2. Insulin resistance causes diabetes and metabolic syndrome
3. Increases protein breakdown
4. Increases fat mass and causes central obesity

You swell all over — fat at the center — develop diabetes, and waste muscle. Imagine a human body that looks like a potato on matchsticks.

Sudden rapid weight gain can be seen when stress overtakes the body.

STARVATION

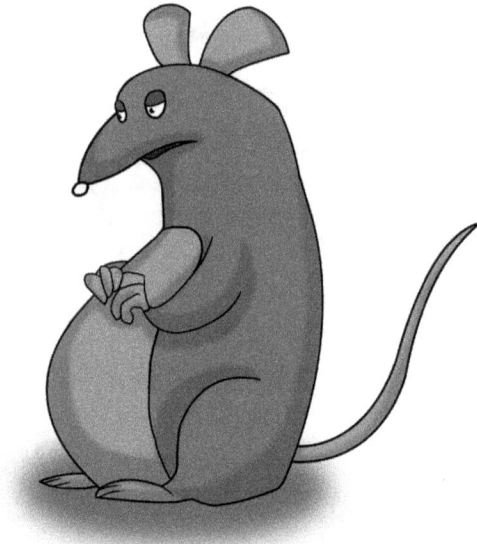

When the human body does not receive energy from eating, it utilizes its glycogen storage, largely stored in muscle. The brain starts utilizing glycogen after six hours of starvation. Usually glycogen storage helps fuel the brain and the body up to 24 hours only. In addition the metabolism shuts down, minimizing calorie expenditure from other parts of the body. This is why if we're starving, our bodies feel tired and we don't feel like being active.

After the glycogen storage is depleted, fat and protein breakdown start to fuel the body's calorie need. Our brain can use only glucose and ketones; fat and protein have to be converted to glucose and ketones in the liver in order for the brain to be able to use calories from these sources. If starvation is prolonged, the body mainly breaks down protein, fueling the body with those calories.

Starvation causes negative effects:

1. Slows down the metabolism
2. Breaks down protein and muscle
3. Causes autophagy, or the self-destruction of cell components, which are less useful for its own survival, hence less energy expenditure
4. Electrolyte imbalances
5. Irregular heart beat
6. Death

SUGAR
Sugar isn't bad, but too much of it at a time is.

The body needs sugar; we can't survive without it (glucose).

Sugar is primarily used by the brain; we need 80-100 grams of sugar a day.

The brain is a control freak; it controls everything, including nutritional intake; body weight; energy levels; and body functions, including the organs responsible for making glucose, breaking down fat or muscle, and yielding energy, as well as which organs will shut down or keep working. The brain craves what it wants; it mostly uses sugar, so it makes you crave sugar. It also deforms and reforms the body, as well as destroys and rebuilds the body.

Sugar can be bad if you consume too much at a time. With too much sugar, the brain alters our normal metabolism, and can make excessive fat.

Imagine your body is in a fluid medium called serum. The serum, is the liquid part of our blood, carries the blood cells and travels all over the body; it reaches your eyes, heart cells, brain cells, kidneys, liver cells — everywhere. When too much sugar goes into the body, the serum, and consequently your organs, begin to be sluggish.

The brain has to ask the pancreas to release the hormone insulin to reduce this sugar level. As we discussed before, the lower levels of insulin in response to not so high sugar levels is very beneficial for body function and glycogen storage. But higher levels of insulin are released in response to higher sugar intake at one time. High insulin levels start turning sugar into fat in short term. Over the long-term, insulin doesn't work very well when there's too much sugar persisting in the system. It starts to get resistance and becomes overwhelmed. It's at this point that you develop diabetes and related insulin-resistance syndromes.

In a hyper-sugar state, the body is negatively impacted with:
1. Chronic inflammation
2. Hardening of the arteries, including heart disease and strokes

3. Uncontrolled diabetes; often with this type of diabetes, you have to use hundreds of units of insulin. It is very labile and hard to control and as compared to traditional diabetes, it is very destructive.

4. As a non-diabetic, 30-60 units of insulin per day is effective, but sometimes in obesity-related diabetes, you need as much as 200-300 units of insulin per day. This is called insulin resistance, and until you lose your central obesity – the fat that accumulates around and inside the belly, this kind of diabetes is difficult to get under control.

5. Accelerated weight gain and obesity

6. Fatty liver – where fat invades the liver.

Essentially, the three S - Starvation, Stress, and (excessive) Sugar...bad, bad, and bad. In todays lives we have plenty of these three as we have so much to do and so little time.

I was excited to see Brenda the next day. I was super careful not to upset her.

First, I told her a rat story. The story goes like this...

What is worse? Stress or fat

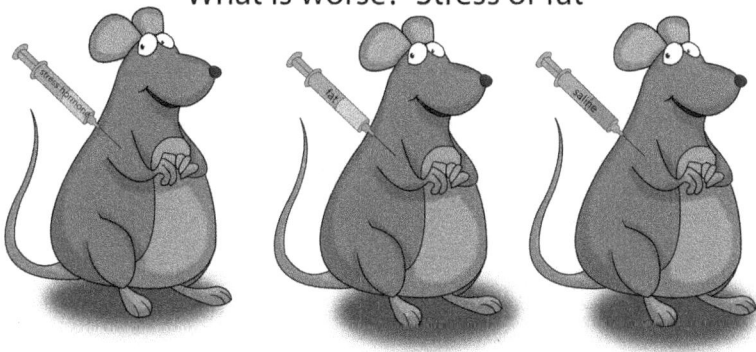

There were three groups of rats in a laboratory. The scientist infused the first group of rats with little doses of adrenalin (stress hormone). Then they infused the second group with little doses of fat droplets. The third group of rats was only infused with saline.

Then the scientists followed the rats. Which group of rats died first?

The rats from the first group (stress hormone-infused) died way ahead of the rats from second (fat-infused), while the third group (saline-infused) lived the longest.

Do you see what stress does to us? Even fat does not kill as fast as stress, though it does kill much more quickly compared to normal (saline-infused) rats.

I taught Brenda how to handle her stress and cut the stress cascade happening in her body. We'll look at this in detail in another chapter.

I gave her three simple tasks as homework.

1. I had her put reminders in her phone, to laugh ten times a day with anything that made her laugh.
   I advised her to do the ten deep-breathing exercises three times a day.
   And I advised her to write down what stressed her.

2. I made her a quiz. She had a basal metabolic rate (BMR) of 1480 calories per day. I asked her to guess which organs and systems spent what percentages of these calories.
   a) Lungs and respiratory system
   b) Heart and circulatory system
   c) Brain and nervous system

d) Stomach and digestive system

e) Muscle and the locomotive system

f) Skin and the sweat/gland system

She guessed that the heart and circulatory system spent the most, but in actuality, the stomach and digestive system spend 30-35% of the calories.

I asked her if she owned a football team, would she rather have her best player sit on the bench, or if she'd prefer him to play his best.

We agreed that he should be in the game, playing to win.

When you chew food, it spends calories. It secretes saliva and digestive juice and carries food down by moving the smooth muscle of the esophagus. It makes digestive enzymes and makes different parts of the gut move. Throughout each of these steps, calories are spent. Every time we eat, we spend calories before we even take in calories.

The idea is to maximize the use of the stomach system, let it work its best to spend calories, and keep the metabolism going quickly.

Brenda said she'd be sure to eat five times a day, in right amounts, to make sure that her stomach system had a chance to work its best.

Eating five times throughout the day assures the brain that you're by no means in starvation mode and that continuous food supplies are guaranteed. This is desirable, as we do not want our brain to look for the calories and start storing them instead of using them.

3. I made her a Fat-Me-Not success plan

I told Brenda to portion control like a pro on every item of food item she eats. She was so happy that she could eat again, that her pizza and bagel weren't off limit.

I told her she could eat everything in the world that God intended us to eat, as long as she stayed within SlimPlate portions.

Brenda was with me as I went through the plan and drew out the steps. I replaced her Mountain Dew with sweetener-free sparkling water.

She happily walked out of the clinic with a drawn-out success plan and the SlimPlate System.

She had a few minor hiccups as a result of bipolar attacks, but aside from that she was well on her way to losing weight. Working with her psychiatrist, we were able to decrease some of her medications, which had been hampering her attempts to lose weight.

In thirteen months, Brenda has lost sixty-seven pounds, and on top of that she's no longer an irritated, easily angered girl. I'm so thrilled to see her progress and dedication.

Though she still has ups and downs and deals with mood instability, she now firmly believes that she can eat and still lose weight.

When you're on the right path, you might encounter some obstacles, but if you keep on going you're sure to reach your goal eventually.

Choose to be on the right path.

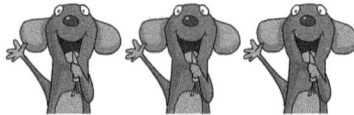

CHAPTER 6
More Extraordinary Stories

More weight loss stories I want everyone to learn from. These are not just stories I am telling. Also hiding behind these stories is something you can use in your own life. So look for it and use it.

Fear and Inflammatory disease

Barbara was a young cute woman who worked in the emergency room at a nearby hospital. She was in her early 30s, with a daughter, a job, and a very supportive father. Unfortunately, she had a bowel disease called Inflammatory Bowel Disease (IBD).

IBD is the disease in which the bowels get intermittently inflamed, so the patient needs to take anti-inflammatory medication (such as steroids). In her short life, she's had to go through a partial bowel resection twice.

Any time Barbara experienced abdominal pain, she had to run to the emergency room. She would get a great deal of work up, including lab work, a CT scan of her abdomen, and repeated treatment with steroids and antibiotics.

As a result, stress, anxiety, and steroid treatment again caused her to gain weight.

There are few diseases that do need intermittent steroid use and that might cause weight gain, and make it difficult to lose weight.

Steroids can reduce bone density, resulting in weak bones.

Steroids can increase insulin resistance and cause diabetes. Nine percent of people on intermittent steroid therapy develop full-blown diabetes.

Steroids can cause fat deposits in various parts of the body, causing obesity.

Steroids can break down muscle and cause muscle atrophy and weakness.

Conditions that may need steroids as part of the treatment include asthma, chronic obstructive pulmonary disease (COPD), rheumatoid arthritis, IBD and many other inflammatory diseases.

Because of this, inflammatory diseases significantly contribute to obesity. Obesity in turn worsens these diseases with increased inflammation.

She had had seventy CT scans and many bouts of steroid treatments. She had also visited the ER about eighty-five times — and she was only thirty-eight years old. She had developed situational depression and was on a number of narcotic pain medications. She was completely unmotivated to improve her life; she had no purpose.

Who wouldn't be depressed, going through the kinds of things Barbara's gone through?

Sometimes life throws everything at you at once.

The one great thing in Barbara's life was her father, who had been with her most of the time she'd been sick.

I had referred her to specialists as a result of continuous and frequent intense pain in her abdomen as well as bouts of diarrhea. This led to more medications, and she kept gaining more weight and getting sicker

We had a long discussion at that point.

1. I advised her to go off all of her pain medications.
2. I also explained to her that she shouldn't go to the ER every time she had pain, and managed to convince her.

As she barely has her gut (after having it resected twice), I explained that she would continue to have diarrhea and discomfort, but that it wasn't so serious that it needs to be treated with strong medications. She even knew what medication she would get in the ER and what the routine would be as she'd been to the ER multiple times.

I asked her why she had gone to the ER so many times. She said that every time she had this pain, she felt like she was dying and that she needed to go to the ER.

I had to reassure her that she wouldn't die from the pain, and advised her that instead, she should come to see me the same day she experienced the pain, or the next morning.

That was the phobia she had built in.

Every time she went to the ER, all eighty-five times, it wasn't that the symptoms of her IBD were flaring up. Less than five times were real disease flare-ups; the rest were a result of her phobia.

Anxiety and phobia make us further damage our bodies. It's a never-ending cycle.

We have to stop the cycle.

1. I advised Barbara that every time she had a pain crisis she should do a non-dairy liquid diet. I planned this out for her and asked her to do specific maneuvers to help ease her pain. I suggested she use a topical pain relief rub as well as a heating pad, and told her to start a journal, so she could write down every time she felt pain and do her best to describe the pain as best she could.

2. I repeatedly reassured and promised her that she wouldn't die from the pain.

She survived the first month without pain medication and realized as a result that she wouldn't die from the pain. Her narcotic pain meds were also worsening her abdominal pain.

Her pain became less severe and she was able to take control of the pain using the above techniques. Her father now controls the medications and fully supports her in going through this process.

This is my favorite part.

I want to share a bit about myself. I am the kind of person who has to see things through to the end. Before I start a project, I always already have the eye to the end.

If I start something, I have to complete it.

We cut the cycle of inflammation from one point. She didn't need to be on any antibiotics or steroids, and very few of the pain medications for a month.

We had to make it stick, what we had achieved so far.

The next task was to deal with the inflammation business arising from the chunk of her belly fat.

Then we met again. Both Barbara and her father were much more hopeful and expectant. Her father brought me the journal Brenda had written in during the past month.

After thoroughly going through the journal, I applauded both of them for what they had done. I explained that with what we had achieved in a month, we had been able to cut the cycle of inflammation from one end.

Both of their eyes sparkled when I said it was time to move to uprooting the inflammation.

Obesity is an inflammatory disease.

1. Obesity worsens inflammation in the body.
2. It impairs the body's immunity and invites more infection.
3. It disturbs the body's healing process.
4. It impairs normal cell growth, causing abnormal growth and cancer.

If Barbara continued with obesity and IBD, her bowel disease would get worse. It would invite multiple gut infections. This is why she was going through multiple rounds of antibiotics. It was definitely delaying her healing and regeneration. If she went on like this, she was likely to get bowel cancer; curability would be very low, as such cancers tend to be highly aggressive. In her case, a premature death would be highly likely; she might not reach the age of fifty.

You might think this is an exaggeration; but we're talking about a 38-year-old woman, with IBD and 140 extra pounds.

Unfortunately, it's a very likely prediction and it is very real and very true.

Obesity was not acknowledged as a disease by the American Medical Association until late 2013.

Obesity-related deaths reported by the CDC reflect far fewer deaths than that actually occur. This is because obesity was not considered as a disease until 2013. This meant cause of death on a death certificate would be something other than obesity, even if obesity was the most pressing reason the disease worsened.

I have many other patients with IBD in my practice that I rarely need to see, but Barbara has the worst kind of IBD.

Her obesity is what makes her IBD the worst kind.

I explained all this to Barbara and her father. They understood it and realized that she needed to lose weight.

So we started her on the Fat-Me-Not success plan.

I suggested she establish a walking habit. Her retired father promised that this would happen.

Walking eases anxiety and stress. It also helps to fight inflammation.

With her bowel problem, Barbara wasn't able to eat many vegetables. She was specifically advised to eat organic meat (to avoid antibiotic manipulated animals) and wholegrain starch (to improve her soluble fiber intake). Many of her vegetable portions were filled with various lentil soups.

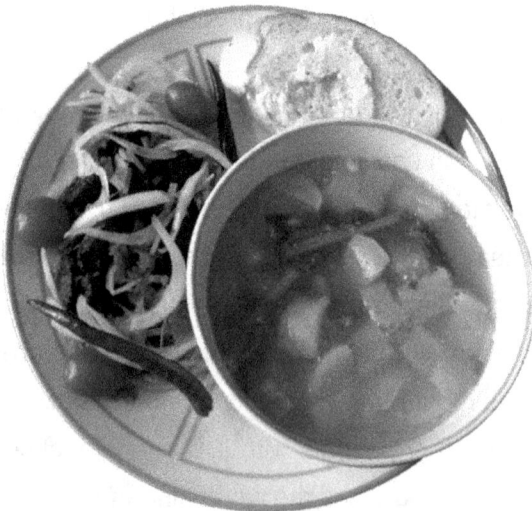

I advised her to fill her meat portion of the SlimPlate with eggs and meat to replenish her vitamin B12; she also received a monthly B12 shot.

Bacteria in the large colon make vitamin B12, but in Barbara's case the bowel there isn't very healthy.

She went through with the success plan; her father motivated her and walked with her daily. Now she walks six miles on a daily basis.

She admitted that walking is her therapist; she doesn't get scare attacks anymore. Barbara is now seventy pounds lighter and has reclaimed her life.

I am incredibly proud of her.

Man and his Manhood: Obesity Induced Low T

Jim is a 45-year-old software engineer. He came to see me after his wife, a 34-year-old primary school teacher, suggested he do so.

His face red, he told me that he was having a problem "getting it up."

As a young, educated man, it was hard, and embarrassing, for him to admit that he couldn't get erection.

Just by looking at him and hearing his complaint, I already knew what his problem was.

It is too common of a problem; I've seen it in many other men, and I've been able to help them.

Jim said that he didn't have any other diseases and that he wasn't on any medications. He admitted that he spent too much time sitting at work and that because of his hectic schedule, most days he didn't get to eat. Barring all that, though, he said that his stress level at work was okay.

So the doctor's big secret is this: even if we know what's going on with our patients, we still go through the questions until the patient is quite sure about what they think.

So I asked Jim a number of questions, including:

Any spontaneous morning erection?

Any decrease in sexual desire?

Any decrease in physical strength?

Any changes in urinary habits, including nighttime frequency of urination, urine stream, or hesitation when urinating?.

Any over-the-counter anabolic steroids or body-building protein powder, bars, or shakes? (Many OTC body-building supplements have the male sex hormone, which can disturb the normal secretion of testosterone from the testes.)

Smoking?

Alcohol use?

Drugs use?

Jim was just a simple workaholic; he was cool with all of the questions.

I asked him what he thought the problem was.

He said he wasn't sure. He said it had started slowly over the last few years, but now he wasn't able to perform sexually at all.

I wrote down a few lab tests and handed him a popular pill prescription (viagra, levitra, cialis).

I explained that I had just bandaged his problem. I asked him to come back and see me in a week, when he could tell me how he had done with the new medication. The goal was to then try to fix the problem.

OBESE MEN WITH SEXUAL DYSFUNCTION, HOW COMMON IT IS?

About 40% of obese men with a BMI of more than 40 have this problem.

Fifty percent of obese men will be diabetics by the time they reach 45 years old.

So I already knew what I would be telling Jim when he returned.

Nothing good comes out of obesity and it is time to take act and take his body back from fat invasion.

Even though Jim hadn't yet suffered from any major diseases, obesity had taken away much of the good things of his youth.

HOW DID IT HAPPEN?

The excess fat tissue secretes estrogen into the blood; it suppresses the hypothalamic-pituitary-adrenal pathway and inhibits the normal secretion of the male hormone testosterone from the testes. This results in a lower level of testosterone in the system, meaning Jim wasn't able to perform the act.

These are the basics of what happens.

OBESITY AND LOW TESTOSTERONE CYCLE

Obesity decreases the testosterone and low testosterone increases central obesity. This is the perfect vicious cycle to become even more obese and with no way to get out of it except by losing weight somehow.

Of the following options, which do you think is the best option to reverse the problem?

A. Viagra, Cialis, Levitra, or other "magic" pills
B. Feed Jim steak and nourishing food
C. Provide him with a love potion 99
D. Testosterone replacement
E. Weight management and testosterone replacement

The answer is E. I knew you'd get it right.

A is only a temporary fix, a Band-Aid over the real problem.

B is a bluff.

C is a joke.

D is incomplete.

E is the correct way to cut the cycle of obesity and poor sex life.

Nearly one in every two obese men has this problem; most of them are under-diagnosed and under- or incompletely treated. Even women have decreased sexual desire from obesity.

Jim came back; this time he had his wife with him. He said he couldn't tolerate the medication as it caused a headache, but that there had been some improvement with the erection.

As expected, his testosterone level was low.

We discussed why this had occurred and the effect it would have on him in the long run.

He understood that he needed to lose weight to cure the problem long-term. So we discussed how he could lose some extra weight.

As we worked through the Fat-Me-Not success plan, he was so excited.

He didn't have to go to a weight-loss meeting.

He didn't have to eat special food.

He really didn't have to put in much effort to lose weight, which was great since he didn't like having to keep buying food in order to lose weight.

One of my weight loss coaches taught Jim and his wife how to use the SlimPlate system. They happily walked out with the SlimPlate set and big smiles.

Jim has lost fifty-five pounds, including his central obesity. He said he and his wife go jogging most of the morning. He eats what his wife puts on the SlimPlate. He takes lunch packed in a box that his wife prepares using the SlimPlate cutter and kit.

He said to me that it was the easiest fifty-five pounds he had ever lost.

I asked Jim if he still felt hungry, as the portions might be less for him.

He said he actually ate less before than what he eats now!

I agree with him. Often, people think obese people eat a lot more than those who don't suffer from obesity in reality, this isn't the case. Something in their eating habit was terribly wrong that made them fat.

Next, we'll discuss eating habits we have and didn't realize that they made us fat.

1. EAT ONE LARGE MEAL A DAY.

This creates fat-saving mode in the body. You might not eat as many total calories, but whatever you do eat will mostly be saved as fat; your body will be preparing for the 20+ hours a day of fasting that results from your eating once a day.

2. NOT EATING BREAKFAST REGULARLY.

I'm a night owl, and I know how precious that last minute of sleep before waking up is. Every day, I jump out of bed, get ready pretty quickly, and then run out of the house with my hair still wet. It dries with the breeze as I drive ☺.

But I always have breakfast, even if I'm in a hurry in the morning. I have a piece of toast with butter spray on it and a cup of tea, or two soft-boiled eggs with a cup of orange juice. You just need three extra minutes to eat breakfast.

Did you know that eating breakfast regularly has many benefits?
- It keeps your metabolism moving quickly.
- It keeps you energetic.
- It reduces morning sluggishness.
- It improves focus at work or school.
- It helps you avoid abnormal eating behaviors like craving and binging.

Basically, it means you start out every day on a healthy path.

3. DRINKING SUGARY DRINKS

Many people don't understand how they can gain weight when they don't eat. What they forget is that the drinks they consume also contain calories. People who don't eat regularly often fall into this category; because they don't eat regularly, their sugar levels go low. As a result, they crave sugar, and people like Jim who are short on time replace food with sugary drinks to keep them going throughout the day.

The end result is that people gain weight without even realizing it.

4. USE DIET SUGARS OR DIET DRINKS

My father is a diabetic. He lives far away in a Southeast Asian country called Burma. Every year, I used to send him packages of diet sugar, and whenever I went to visit him I carried it with me.

My father hangs out with his friends, most of whom were diabetics. I became a major supplier of diet sugar for them, buying in bulk and supplying them regularly. I bought diet sugar for them to use in baking and coffee, as well as individual packages to carry along with them to their coffee shops.

Back then, that was what we thought we needed to do for diabetic patients.

After I started my medical practice, I saw many young patients come in with headaches, fogginess, and inability to focus, as well as sweet-cravings and other symptoms.

I looked into the literature and found many side effects. I also unexpectedly discovered that artificial sweetener users faced many of these problems.

There was research done on artificial sweeteners that suggested that people actually ate 40% more sugar after consuming diet drinks when compared to regular drinks.

The brain and circulating red blood cells mainly use sugar (glucose) for energy. We're depriving ourselves of sugar when we use an artificial sweetener, which means that the brain craves sugar for more energy.

I want to clarify one thing. Artificial sweeteners are bad not because of the word 'artificial' in the name, but because of the way they act on our bodies. They give us the taste of sugar without providing the calories that we need. It teases the brain in a bad way.

Marketers realized that people didn't like the sound of "artificial", so they started using "natural" instead, so that people think it's safe to take.

But if natural sweeteners only give the sweet taste without the calories, then it's just as bad as artificial sweeteners.

I advise my patients to throw away the sweeteners.

Essentially, artificial sweeteners make chaos of your metabolism when you're trying to lose weight.

Even for diabetic patients, I suggest that they use regular sugar — just in limited portions.

My father and his friends drink four cups of tea a day. I advised them to use a half of a SlimPlate mug each time, using regular crystal sugar and cream. I no longer provide them with artificial sweeteners.

5. EAT INFREQUENTLY OR SKIP MEALS

Everyone experiences the feeling of not having enough time. This causes us to eat less frequently and skip meals.

Our bodies store calories in the short-term as glycogen; this store usually serves the body's needs for six to twelve hours. Between mealtimes, the glycogen slowly depletes; the brain begins to shut down its energy-spending system and slow down the metabolism. But if the food intake is not regular and your body is not sure when it will get it next, it will start storing your food as fat rather than glycogen. That is because fat is a long term storage.

Unnecessary Surgery: The right thing to do?

I met Brittany in the office one day.

She was a 22-year-old college student. She came in to see me and announced that she wanted her gallbladder removed.

I asked if she had abdominal pain or nausea or any other symptoms.

Brittany told me that she was going to a foreign country to study for few years and that before she left, she wanted her gall-bladder removed.

She said that her mother's gallbladder was resected when she was twenty-eight; her older sister had had gallbladder resection the previous year, at age twenty-three. And her younger sister, at age nineteen, had also gone through gallbladder resection. Brittany said that she was going to go through the same thing soon, and that she didn't want to go through it in a foreign country.

I probed further and discovered that she had no complaints of abdominal pain, bloating, nausea, or vomiting, but that she had occasional heartburn.

She didn't have any of the symptoms of gallbladder inflammation disease, but was convinced she was going to get it eventually, and didn't want that to happen abroad.

I paused for a moment to think about how to answer that. What she said was right; I agreed that she would eventually suffer from an inflamed gallbladder and would need to go through surgery like her sisters did.

I couldn't tell her to have the surgery as she didn't have the disease, but she was right that she had a high chance of getting gallbladder disease, making it possible that it would become a problem while abroad.

At the same time, Brittany's gallbladder hadn't yet shown any signs of illness; letting her go through the surgery wouldn't be right. Any procedure or surgery must be medically necessary, as there is always a possibility of life-threatening complications, regardless of how non-invasive the procedure is.

GALLBLADDER, ACID REFLUX, AND FATTY LIVER DISEASE IN THE OBESE POPULATION

Gallstones and inflammation of the gallbladder highly correlates with body weight. The higher your body weight, the more likely that you will get inflammatory gallbladder disease. If you have a BMI of 30, the odds are 3.7% higher; if your BMI is 40, the odds are doubled 7.5% higher. Sixty percent of people suffer from NASH (fatty liver –alcoholic liver without drinking alcohol).

If a gallbladder attack strikes, you'll suffer from abdominal pain, nausea, and vomiting, and ultimately may be admitted to the hospital for gallbladder resection surgery. Gallbladder resection may have long-term consequences such as indigestion, mal-absorption, and chronic diarrhea.

I explained to Brittany that we shouldn't take out her gallbladder and what we were going to do to protect it so that it wouldn't need to be removed.

Gallbladder disease is common in women who are obese, sedentary, and use contraceptive pills. As Brittany had a strong family history, her risk was even higher.

There are many other risk factors to gallbladder disease.

We discussed how we were going to tackle the gallbladder attacks. I advised her to:

1. Lose weight and keep it down
2. Use non-estrogen based contraceptive
3. Increase her physical activity

She was enthusiastic about this plan. Her mother was also happy, and was cheering Brittany on her attempt to lose weight.

By improving her lifestyle to lose weight and by making medication changes, Brittany started on her weight-loss journey.

She joined our weight-loss boot camp program and went through the first three months before going abroad. She lost thirty-two pounds. She is a softball player and she played actively during her journey.

She was watched closely due to her rapid weight loss, as that in turn could potentially cause gallstone diseases, too. She was put on bile salt therapy for the prevention of gallbladder disease.

It has been few years now. I continue to see Brittany's family; they tell me how well she's doing with her studies. To date, she has not suffered from any gallstone diseases.

Am I sure that she won't need a gallbladder surgery in the future?

I can't be one hundred percent sure that Brittany will never need gallbladder surgery, but I do know that the action we took was the right thing to do for that situation. Brittany was able to eliminate everything that put her at risk for this kind of disease, and as a result she has been able to live the last several years without needing surgery and a healthier active life.

One of the many benefits of staying lean is that you need less medical procedures, which is always a good thing.

Rashes and Crashes

Daytona was a gorgeous, fun-loving girl; she's always laughing. But she had a little secret.

One day, she asked me to write her a letter of medical necessity to permit her to bring a personal fan to her class.

As I was typing the letter, she explained that she had a weird skin problem. She told me that if she sweated in class, she had to run to the bathroom, take off her clothes, and fan the area to cool it down. Otherwise, she would tear her skin to shreds because it itched so badly.

I said to her that it sounded like a serious problem, asked her how long she'd had it, and asked her to show me.

She showed me the inner part of her groin and genital areas and her under-breast area. Excoriated, angry-looking, red, and raw skin told me the intensity of the problem. Different patches of dry, dark brown areas and red, wet, raw areas told me that she had had this repeatedly and that it was a recurring problem.

I took samples to send for cultures, including fungal infections.

I asked her several other questions, including what perfume, deodorant, and chemical soap she used.

I found out that she tended to get oral thrush and yeast infections in her toenails.

She thought they were okay; she just used over-the-counter medications with gold bond and used nail polish to cover up the problem.

She admitted that she had vaginal yeast infections after most of her periods and that she used over-the-counter medication.

She had started out laughing about it, but as she went on talking, the laughter faded and she began to cry.

She said she was very shy about her patchy skin discoloration and all these itches; she hadn't felt confident to date anyone.

I assured her that it wasn't an incurable disease and that we could treat it.

She said she had seen many doctors, including specialists like gynecologists and dermatologists, and they had prescribed her many medications. She was able to tell me everything that she had used and how they had helped her for a short period of time before the problem came back.

She was basically able to recite every medication that can be used for this condition.

I told her that it was bound to come back, because there was one thing she hadn't tried yet.

She was excited. She told me that whatever it was, she would get it, would do it, would take it, because her skin condition was really bothering her.

I explained to her that her skin lesions had originally started as friction; they then got infected with yeast before being superinfected by secondary bacterial infections. She had friction all over her body, including under her arms, breasts, and abdominal folds, and around her groin.

To make matters worse, her cutaneous yeast infection had spread to the oral cavity and vaginal mucosa.

Yeast is slow growing and very annoying to get rid of. Yeast likes moisture and tends to hang around where the moisture is. This is why you find yeast under toenails when we sweat in our socks.

Yeast is more common in people with obesity as these people have a thicker fat layer and multiple skin folds that cause friction, interrupting skin integrity. Increased sweating creates a moist and damp environment that makes a very inviting environment for infections. Obese people's skin also has less collagen as a result of the excess fat, which decreases circulation and disrupts normal skin healing.

It's a bad combination. We see how the cause, aggravation, and the impaired healing provide the foundation for Daytona's notorious, recurrent skin infection.

The answer, as you know by now, was for Daytona to lose weight: to lose the excessive fat folds.
1. I took a few samples and gave her some guidelines to follow, including: Shower twice daily with mild soap.
2. Don't use tampons; use feminine pads instead.
3. Don't use chemical deodorants or perfumes.
4. Wash up immediately if you sweat excessively.
5. Rinse your mouth with salt water after every meal.
6. Change your socks at least twice daily. If you sweat, change them again.
7. Use loose cotton undergarments.
8. Avoid nail salons.

9. Keep all old shoes under the sun and treat them for mold.

10. Avoid repeat infections by not wearing moldy shoes.

11. Avoid use of antibiotics unless absolutely necessary.

Daytona joined our weight-loss boot camp and began her weight-loss journey. She gave up diet and sugary drinks completely.

Yeast and bacteria really like sugar in the body.

Daytona was getting multiple antibiotics for rotating infections in different parts of her body. This disrupted her body's entire defense mechanism, reducing her ability to fight infection.

Now, Daytona is a happy girl; she laughs constantly. She no longer needs her personal fan. Forty-two pounds lighter, and she's declared her victory over her infections.

Remember, you can't just cover up a condition. You have to dig it out from the root.

When the doctor says that you need to lose weight, don't take it lightly. Don't just agree and then do nothing. You cannot even imagine how many problems you face everyday can just go away after losing weight.

Act on it.

Losing weight is the most powerful thing you can do to lead a better life. I wouldn't take one billion dollars in exchange for obesity. Staying lean is more powerful than any sum of money.

Obesity and the risk of cancer

Obesity can increase the risk of cancer by up to 40%.

Common cancers related to obesity include:

- Breast cancer
- Uterus cancer
- Ovarian cancer
- Cervical cancer
- Colon cancer
- Esophageal cancer
- Pancreatic cancer
- Stomach cancer
- Liver cancer
- Kidney cancer
- Prostate cancer

A Diagnosis Delayed

Natasha was a morbidly obese, 37-year-old woman; she weighed close to 400 pounds. I looked after her as a medical doctor in the hospital, where she was admitted for long-standing and complicated medical problems five years ago.

Her complaint was persistent nausea. She went through multiple diagnostic tests, including endoscopy, ultrasound, and a CAT scan of the abdomen. Multiple specialists followed her case in the hospital.

We couldn't find a reason for her persistent nausea and vomiting, so we decided to do an MRI of her abdomen to see what we could find.

The problem was that Natasha couldn't fit in the hospital MRI machine. And because of her excessive fatty tissue, the results of the ultrasounds and CAT scans were also unclear; repeating the tests wouldn't yield any more information.

We put our heads together to figure out how to reach a diagnosis. This was the first time I had ever experienced this kind of situation.

Then, one doctor came up with the idea of using the bigger MRI machine at the regional zoo. Because it was used to scan elephants and other large animals, it was capable of fitting someone with a larger body size.

We discussed this possibility with Natasha and her family and, with their agreement and permission, we contacted the zoo. As the machine had previously been used for animals, it took a while to get it ready to use it on a person. Once the zoo had completed its preparations, Natasha was transferred and the MRI was completed.

The MRI showed pancreatic cancer that had spread to the liver.

Natasha was only 37 years old. The situation seemed unreal, but unfortunately for Natasha, it was very real.

Natasha passed away a few months after her diagnosis.

What did we learn from Natasha's condition, aside from the fact that it brings sadness and loss?

- Obesity can be very dangerous.
- Obesity can delay diagnosis.
- Obesity can make it impossible for diagnostic tests to be useful.

Did you know:

1. We can't replace a knee or hip if the patient is very obese; the individual has to live in pain or sedating pain medication until they die, because prosthetic knees have weight limits.
2. If a patient is very obese, we can't fix the spine; the individual has to live under heavy pain medicine and drowsiness from it until obesity, or something else, kills them.
3. We can't use the traditional diagnostic tests on morbidly obese people, meaning that diagnosis, and treatment get delayed and can result in a loss of life.
4. Obesity resists conventional treatment.
5. Diseases are worse for individuals suffering from obesity than for those who are not obese.

Yet despite this, I see people carrying above 300 pounds every day unaware of the risks they face.

I've told you these stories so that you can understand how obesity affects our bodies.

Often, primary care doctors tell their patients that they need to lose weight, but this doesn't seem to sink in.

Even I hesitate to tell to my patients that they need to lose weight, as it can be a sensitive topic and I don't like to upset them.

As you can see from the above stories, I often wait for my patients to tell me what their problems are first.

I'm an Asian immigrant, and there are many cultural differences between the US and Asian countries. For instance, in Asian countries, the people that are close to you will tell you if you've become fat. They won't sugarcoat it; they'll bluntly tell you that you've put on weight, that you're fat and need to do something about it.

It isn't that they're rude; it's a way of showing care about another person. They take on other people's problems as their own.

Here in the US, on the other hand, we are respectful of individual privacy and consider weight issues to be personal and private.

Often my obese patients have no idea how much they weigh; they have avoided looking in the mirror in months, or haven't seen their whole body in a mirror for years.

Even if someone says that they're overweight, the culturally expected, appropriate response is to tell the person that they look fine, whether you think that that's the case or not.

Many doctors know that a patient is obese, but they still chose not to mention it.

As a result, many people simply think they don't need to lose weight, much less realize that they are overweight or obese.

I will give you a rough guide for planning your weight loss journey. This can change based on your height.

Generally speaking, for women:

- If your weight reaches 160 pounds, make plans to lose weight.
- If your weight reaches 180 pounds, start your weight-loss journey immediately.
- If your weight reaches 230 pounds, you need to be on a weight loss program that works well for you so that you can start seeing your weight go down sooner rather than later.
- If your weight reaches 250 pounds, seek additional professional help.
- If your weight reaches 300 pounds, you should consult a doctor about possible surgical options or putting a serious weight loss plan in place in order to lose weight.

Generally speaking, for men:

- If your weight reaches 200 pounds, make plans to lose weight.
- If your weight reaches 220 pounds, start your weight-loss journey immediately.
- If your weight reaches 250 pounds, you need to be on an effective weight loss program so that you can start seeing your weight go down sooner rather than later.
- If your weight reaches 280 pounds, seek additional professional help.
- If your weight reaches 320 pounds, you should consult a doctor about possible surgical options or putting a serious weight loss plan in place in order to lose weight.

Make your decision according to where your weight currently is. Also factor in your height and talk to your doctor about your weight.

Obesity and good health can't coexist; you can either have one or the other. Just having normal labs dos not mean one is healthy.

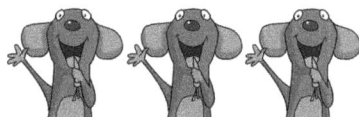

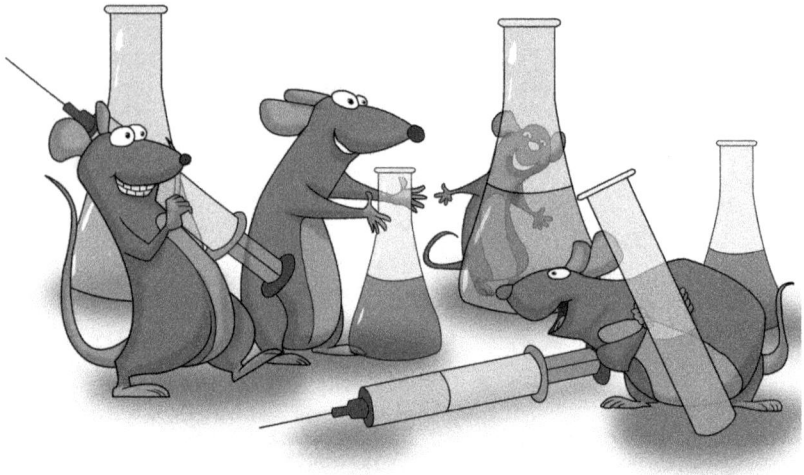

Chapter 7
Ratz Stories

Cutting Edge Weight Loss Research Made Simple

Ratz Stories: Cutting Edge Weight Loss Research Made Simple

I remember one Monday when I returned to work after recovering from a cold. It was one of those times when the cold weather had hit the state hard and many people were sick. I wasn't the only one coughing; my patients were coughing as well.

A patient asked me what I was taking for my cough. I smiled beneath my facemask and told her, jokingly, that I couldn't give her my magic cough syrup.

The truth is, I can't give my patients the remedy I use for a cough. I use warm honey — I use a chopstick tip dipped in warm honey to calm my throat. It works for me.

Just because I've used that remedy, I can't recommend that others use it to treat their cough.

This is because warm honey hasn't been proven to be efficacious or safe, and its proper use has not been studied.

My point here is that though I might personally use something to soothe my throat, I can't recommend something that hasn't been scientifically studied and that isn't medically sound to my patients.

This is a chapter related to the latest science behind obesity and weight loss treatment. The diets we hear nowadays have been discovered in the 1960s. That is old research. My aim to write this book is to introduce you to the cutting edge research that is redefining how to lose weight and treat obesity. We are finding that losing weight is way simpler than we earlier thought. Also the deprivation diets like low fat diet, low carb diets are doing more harm than good when it comes to sustaining weight loss.

So we will talk about Ratz. With Ratz I mean the mice, the rats, the hamsters who toil in the laboratories giving us answers about our own body. Most of the mice studied in laboratories are DIO (Diet Induced Obese) mice; the chapter is therefore called "Ratz Stories" in honor of the mice sacrificed to gain medical knowledge to help mankind.

The medicine I practice always has scientific efficacy, safety, well-accepted guidelines, and well-researched techniques.

There is a large gap between current scientific research findings and current weight-loss products on the market.

This chapter aims to make this gap smaller by providing easy explanations of complicated current research findings for you. In fact it will make it very easy for you to understand the research.

My hope is that you will therefore be able to understand the biologically correct choices to make for your body. With this knowledge, you will be able to avoid products marketed for weight-loss that might actually cause harm.

Some of the research is very technical, but this chapter will simplify it so that it's easy to understand and you don't feel like you are attending a medical school.

Research Study: Why portion control? What Ratz taught us?

GASTRIC BYPASS SURGERY: THE RESULTS EXPLAINED

So far, gastric bypass surgery has proven to be the most effective (and extreme) weight loss method, albeit most dangerous one too.

We know it isn't possible for everyone who needs to lose weight to go through gastric bypass surgery. The question, therefore, is whether we can achieve similar weight loss without going through surgery.

To learn how this is possible, we're going to look at a new research study in which the effects of gastric bypass surgery was tested on mice.

PROCESS OF GASTRIC BYPASS

After gastric bypass, patients are unable to eat large amounts of food at once; this means they eat smaller meals more frequently. Previously, researchers thought the reason the surgery was effective was this limited intake of food by surgically reducing the size of the stomach.

However, that is no longer holds true.

Researchers discovered that there is a change in our body after gastric bypass surgery that causes weight loss. There is a change in the gastric hormones and the bacterial flora that lives in the gut.

Interestingly enough, this is what we learnt from the research study on mice. So here is what they did.

The first group of obese mice went through gastric bypass surgery and lost weight.

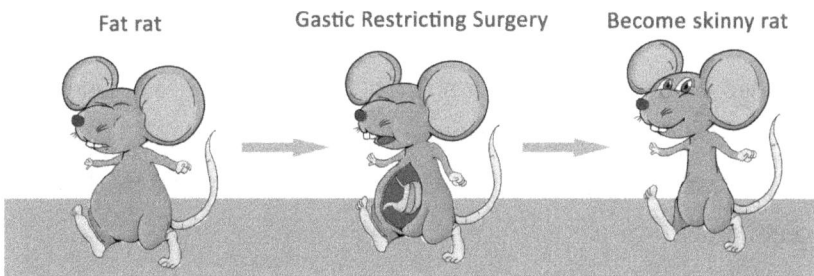

Fat rat   Gastic Restricting Surgery   Become skinny rat

The second group of obese mice was given the bacterial flora (bacteria from the stomach) from the first group. The weight loss that resulted in this second group was the same as that of the first, even though the second group didn't go through the surgery.

As a result, researchers thought that the change of bacteria must have been causing the weight loss. The question, then, was why the bacteria had changed. Did the surgery cause the change? Or was it a result of smaller stomach and portioning?

Without any clear answers, the researchers continued their study with two more groups of mice.

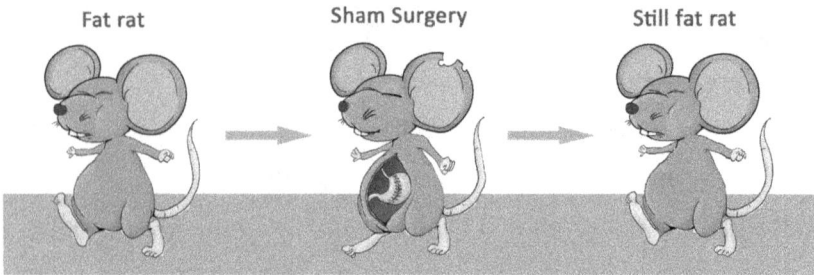

Fat rat   Sham Surgery   Still fat rat

The third group of obese mice was given a sham surgery. This is when a gastric bypass surgery is done, but, as shown in the above picture, everything is re-sutured. There is no actual portioning of the stomach, as it remains exactly the same size.

The fourth group of obese mice was given the bacterial flora from the third group following their sham surgery, just as the researchers had done with the first two groups.

The result? There was no weight loss in either the third or the fourth group.

Voila! Portioning the stomach helps with losing weight, possibly due to all of the beneficial changes in the gut's hormone and flora.

Gastric surgery changes the gut hormones and bacterial flora, resulting in effective weight loss. So somehow the bacteria in our gut are controlling our weight. Creepy but we will learn that later how.

> *Bottom Line: Portioning food before you eat is safer than portioning the stomach.*

Research Study: What is brown fat? How does it affect weight loss?

Our body has two types of fat, namely the white fat and the brown fat. Brown fat is a type of fat that has many mitochondria — the tiniest energizing batteries in the cell. This is a good kind of fat and the kind of fat you want in your body. Brown fat actually burns excessive unwanted fat, also known as white fat.

Think of brown fat like muscle. It promotes energy expenditure and burns off unwanted fat. Brown fat promotes thermogenesis, mitochondrial energetics, and energy expenditure, and also protects from diabetes and obesity.

So now scientists are looking into how to change white fat to brown fat in the body in order to use this as a way to lose the unwanted fat and thus lose weight.

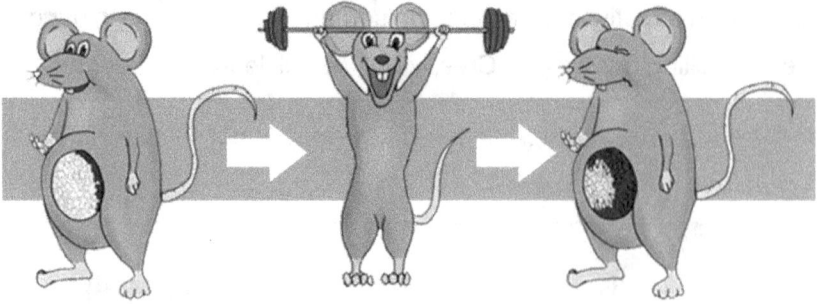

Research shows that exercising more often could transform unwanted white fat cells into the more desirable brown fat.

There is an interesting study that has been done on mice. When the scientists activated a gene in Mr. Ratz to produce more Irisin – a hormone released by our muscles, Mr, Ratz started turning its white fat into brown fat and started losing weight. This study tells us that we might actually be able to change the white fat we have into the brown fat we want.

What does that mean? It means we can lose the unwanted fat easier by converting it into brown fat and therefore lose weight.

There are few things capable of transforming white fat to brown. One of them is Irisin, the hormone produced by muscle which was used in this research study.

Irisin is a muscle hormone that increases with exercise and general activity and building muscles.

Essentially, this study tells us to exercise more. The more active you are, the more you will brown your white fat, improve your metabolism, and lose weight.

> *Bottom Line: Thirty minutes of physical activity (any activity that makes you sweat counts) will make your weight loss journey easier. So choose something fun for you to do that makes you sweat and adopt that practice daily. Also work on increasing your muscle mass so don't ignore strength training and do just aerobics.*

Personally, I like hula hooping and dancing (like nobody is watching me). Twice a week, I give myself a challenge program. You can also choose your favorite challenge program from the SlimPlate System exercise videos available through our mobile app, or subscribe to our YouTube channel. It is available free to anyone.

Research Study: Eating behaviors that we learn from Ratz

SUGARY DRINKS CAUSE BINGE EATING AND FOOD ADDICTION

The laboratory mice Mr. Ratz were given a sugary liquid comparable to the amount of sugar found in an average soda. When Mr. Ratz was given this sugar solution, he would eat more than usual in the first hour.

The amount Mr. Ratz eats was recorded. As the days went on, it became clear that he was eating more and more, proving his binge-eating behavior triggered by sugary drinks. This behavior carried on for a long time even after the sugary drinks were stopped.

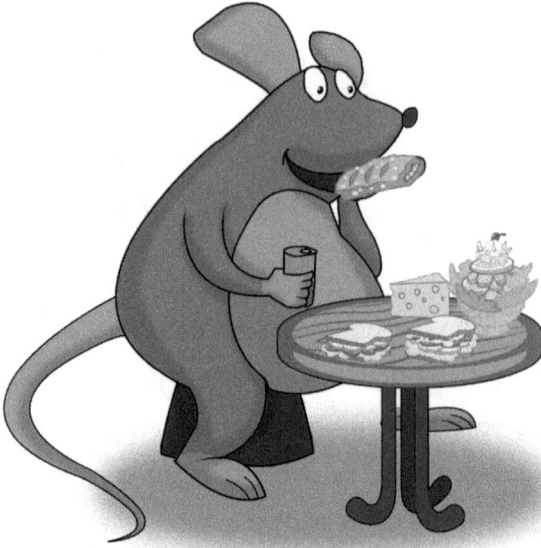

Fat causing binge eating

When a well-fed Mr. Ratz was given access to shortening (vegetable fat), he binged on his food in first hour following eating as well.

FAT AND SUGAR TOGETHER (LIKE A COOKIE OR PIECE OF CAKE)

When Mr. Ratz was fed a mixture of fat and sugar, the rat binges so much that it can consume more than half of their daily calorie requirement within a two-hour period.

FOOD ADDICTION

After being given sugary drinks, food was withheld from Mr. Ratz for twenty-four hours. He went into withdrawal. His teeth chattered, his forepaws trembled, and he suffered from head shaking. He wanted his soda.

When food was withheld, he kept running to press a lever to get his soda.

As researchers learn about binging and addiction in animals, they begin to study how humans show their addiction to food. There is an addiction center in the brain, and researchers have done special scans of the brains of obese individuals.

The brain scan (Positron Emission Tomography (PET) scan) signals that food addiction is identical to drug addiction.

Essentially, abnormal eating behaviors like binge eating, cravings, and addiction exist and are caused by an individual's food choices.

Bottom Line: If you decide to eat that cookie, cake or pastry now, it won't satisfy your craving. It will make it worse and you will be craving for rest of the day or more.

Points to remember!
1. Low carb diets (which become high fat diets) are not a healthy way to lose weight; you develop abnormal eating behaviors and can never reach a goal of long-term weight-loss.
2. Low fat diets (which become high carb diets) can cause binging and addiction and can land you in a never-ending weight-loss/weight gain cycle as you lose your eating signals and controls.
3. The success of long-term weight-loss is in a balanced diet.
4. Drink a glass of water when you consume your meals. With breakfast, you can drink coffee, tea, or juice.

Research Study: Premature ovarian failure, infertility and obesity

This time, the mice were put in three groups.

The first group was fed normally.

The second was fed 70% less than normal.

The third group was given a high fat diet.

The groups were observed over many months. The mice in the third group were found to weigh more. They were also centrally obese and suffered from larger ovaries. When analyzing the ovaries of this third group, they saw that there were fewer healthy ovarian follicles and that a greater number had atretic (shrunk) follicles.

Obese women are at high risk of losing their fertility due to the loss of so many ovarian follicles; they are also at a higher risk of premature ovarian failure.

You can see high fat diet can make you gain weight and also cause fertility problem. Again low carb diet usually ends up being a high fat diet because of choice of foods so low carb diet is not a good idea. If you decide to go low fat and low carb diet then you don't have much left to eat. That is why a balanced diet is important for weight loss.

> *Bottom Line: Obesity can cause infertility.*

Research Study: High fat diet - Causing our brains to inflame

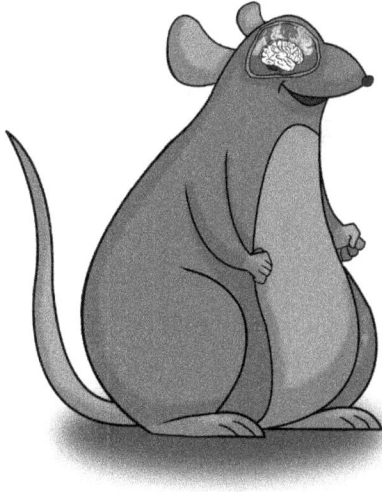

I have always advised my patients to eat a well-balance diet.

We can see another reason to do this in the following story.

Mice were put into two groups, which were fed with a moderate fat diet. The differences in the diets were in the saturated fat, as one group received a diet consisting of 60% saturated fat (butter) and the other only 20% saturated fat (coconut oil). Then the animals were sacrificed and their brains were analyzed. The brains of the butter-fed Mr. Ratz were filled with inflammation and inflammatory chemicals.

> *Bottom Line: Obesity is an overwhelming inflammatory disease. Inflammatory signals creep over the entire body and cause multiple diseases.*

When I was in medical school, one of the teachers, who is well-known for his ability to diagnose diseases, shared his secret with us. He told us that if you see tiger stripes, you're probably looking at a tiger. It can't be a zebra, cat, lion, and tiger all combined in one body.

Sometimes in medicine, things can be vague and confusing, but a single body can't have multiple medical problems. Instead, as doctors our job is to find a single root to all of the problems, which will usually lead us to the most likely diagnosis.

Nowadays, an individual patient can have diabetes, heart disease, sleep apnea, severe arthritis, fatty liver, and gallbladder disease in a single body. If we see many overwhelming diseases like this, we know that obesity is the culprit. The root problem causing all of these sicknesses is obesity aka fat mass and sick inflamed fat tissue.

Obesity can destroy all or many different parts of our body just like a cancer can destroy.

Research Study: Mr. Ratz and the balloon in his stomach

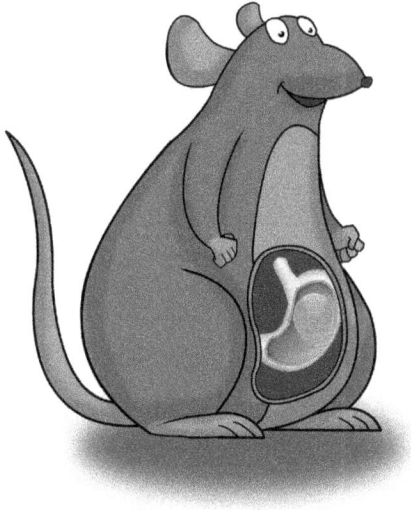

Next we will talk about mimicking the gastric restriction (portioning) study in Mr. Ratz

It is multi-steps studies and I am breaking it down to make it easy to follow.

A gastric balloon was placed in Mr. Ratz's stomach, non-surgically. The researchers followed his progress and found that over the course of the next two months, Mr. Ratz was eating less and less. After two months, the balloon was removed, allowing Mr. Ratz to eat without the balloon inflation. The result was that Mr. Ratz lost a lot of weight when the balloon was in place, and that further, once the balloon was removed, he was able to maintain that weight loss.

Stomach restriction is very effective for losing weight. The mice were able to maintain their reduced weight, as they had been trained over the course of eight weeks to be used to the limited stomach portion.

> *Bottom Line: It is not the stomach size that makes you eat less. Remember the mice were eating less even after the balloon was removed. So you can train your stomach to ask for less.*

Research Study: Humans and the balloon in their stomachs

Following the above study, the scientists stepped up to studying humans.

A gastric balloon was inserted into both lean and obese subjects. The balloons were inflated with water via a tube that was left in place. 200ml, 400ml, 600ml, and 800ml were inserted on different days before meals. The result was that as the gastric balloon was inflated with more water, people ate up to 40% less.

In this human study the gastric balloon inflation was directly related to weight loss; results were seen as soon as the first week.

I advised my patients to develop the habit of drinking a cup of water before and after meals as well as with snacks. This is the easiest way to portion the stomach.

There have been other studies done in Asians (Koreans And Japanese) subjects in which individuals drink a cup of thin soup or hot, unsweetened tea with their meals. This may partly explain why they are the leanest people in the world.

In another subsequent study, balloons in human subjects were inflated with 250ml and 500ml of liquid. At the same time, the brain was scanned with an MRI in order to study the different areas of the brain. This allowed scientists to see which parts of the brain were activated while the stomach was distended.

The area of the brain related to the reward and emotion center of the brain (the amygdala, or craving center) was activated. Amygdala activation relates to weight loss.

So the stomach is distended and the amygdala is activated; this may result the ultimate weight loss.

In another study on eating behavior, both lean and obese human subjects were stimulated by the sight and smell of high-energy, dense (fatty) food vs. low-energy, dense (protein or carb) food.

As they were being teased with this sight and smell, their heads were scanned by an MRI.

The reward center area of the brain was activated more strongly for fatty food in obese people than in lean people.

If we eat too much fatty food, we have the incessant desire to eat even if we're not hungry; this makes it easier to stimulate obese people.

Another study, on eating behavior pre- and post-bariatric surgery, analyzed food cues with fatty foods versus protein or carbs, as in the above study. Brain scan analysis showed that before the surgery, abnormal eating behaviors were noted, and then after the surgery this was normalized and reversed in the same patients.

POINTS

- The amount of food we eat determines our weight.
- The food we eat also affects our eating behavior; fatty foods make us eat more, while leaner foods make us eat less.
- Fatty foods make us eat more even if we aren't hungry, a symptom of food addiction.
- These abnormal eating behaviors can be reversed when you begin eating correctly: the right food in the right proportions.

Bottom Line: What you eat and how much you eat decides what you will eat and how much you will eat in the future. So to break this cycle you have to start eating right and every thing else will fall into place.

Research Study: The effect of HCG injections on weight loss: "None exists"

In one study, researchers created four groups, as seen below:

Obese Ratz	Lean Ratz
1. HCG shot	3. HCG shot
2. No HCG shot	4. No HCG shot

The fat tissues were evaluated under the microscope; multiple other analyses were undertaken on changes in these groups at the ultra-structural level.

No microscopic changes that could account for fat loss were noted in the HCG shot groups or the control (non-HCG) groups.

If the HCG shots were efficacious for losing weight, we would see dissolution of fat in the obese Mr. Ratz.

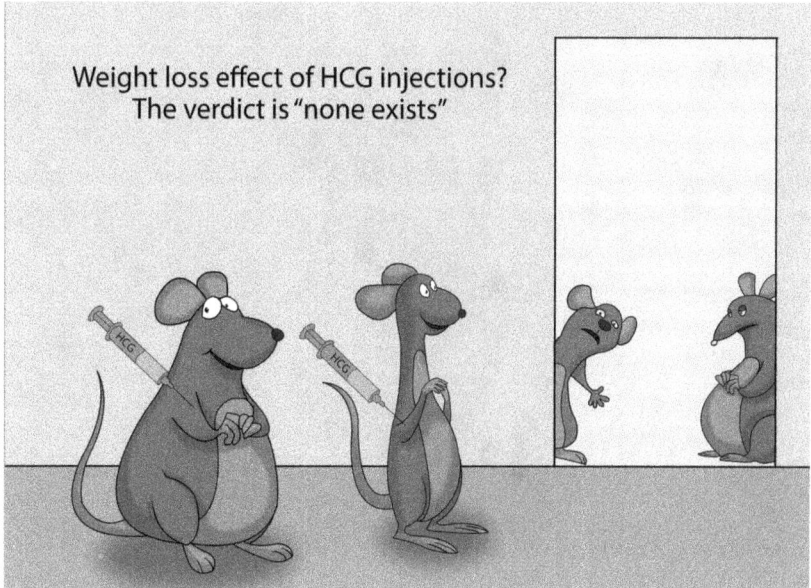

Weight loss effect of HCG injections?
The verdict is "none exists"

Many other human studies have shown that the HCG shots do not offer additional weight loss than does the restricted diet that accompanies it. When you get the HCG shot, it is accompanied either by a low-calorie or a high-protein diet. The reason people lose weight in HCG clinics is not because of the HCG shot, but instead because of the diet they are on.

Not only are HCG shots ineffective, but they can also be dangerous. Life-threatening complications related to HCG have been reported, including blood clots in the body, legs, and lungs.

Research Study: High protein diets and their benefits

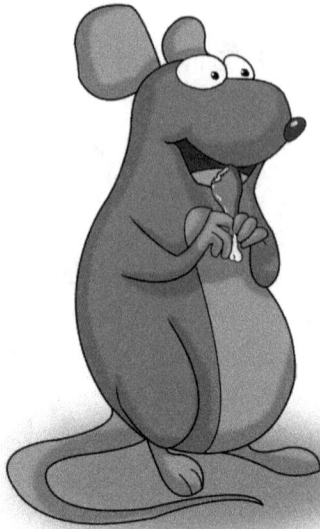

High-protein diets can promote weight loss and weight maintenance in both animals and humans. In addition, high-protein diets have the potential to improve glucose homeostasis, increase energy expenditure (EE), lower blood lipids, reduce blood pressure, and preserve lean body mass.

This time, Mr. Ratz was fed with a high-protein diet (50% protein). Mr. Ratz had been previously checked on glucose control and calorie consumption.

The result was that after the high-protein diet, their sugar control was much better and they spent more calories than before.

This was confirmed in pigs and other mammals as well as in human subjects.

BENEFITS OF A HIGH PROTEIN DIET

1. Increase energy expenditure
2. Increase satiety
3. Higher water intake
4. Modest glucose control improvement
5. Modest cholesterol improvement
6. Modest improvement in blood pressure control (5-10mmhg)

In a subsequent study, one group was given a high-protein diet (50%) while the other was given an appropriate-protein diet (10%).

1. The study found that: A high-protein diet can increase water intake by 50-75% compared to an appropriate-protein diet.
2. It was reported that by drinking more water, metabolic rates could be increased by 30%.
3. A high-protein diet can reduce the fat content of the fatty liver by 50% more when compared to an appropriate-protein diet.

> *Bottom Line: Eat more proteins to lose weight.*

I would like to mention few of the scientific studies have also proven the benefits of drinking water. We will not go in the details of these studies but here are the benefits of drinking water.

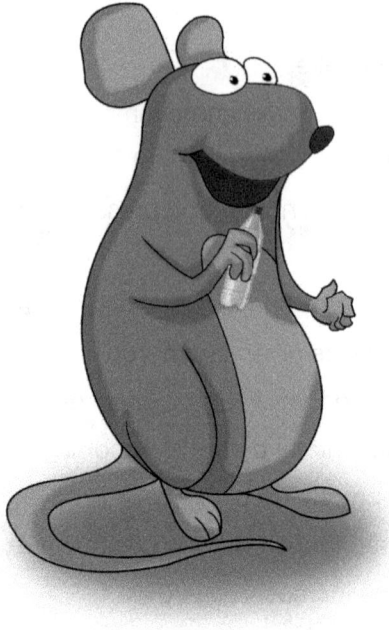

1. Lower energy intake
2. Facilitate long-term weight loss
3. Effectively reduce weight gain
4. Increase metabolic rate by stimulating sympathetic systems
5. Regulate the metabolism with water
6. Improves the exercise capacity of muscle

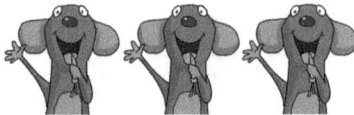

Chapter 8

Why Diet Trumps Exercise?

How The Bacteria in Our Gut is Hacking Our Nervous System and Controlling What We Eat and What We Weigh.

Diet Trumps Exercise

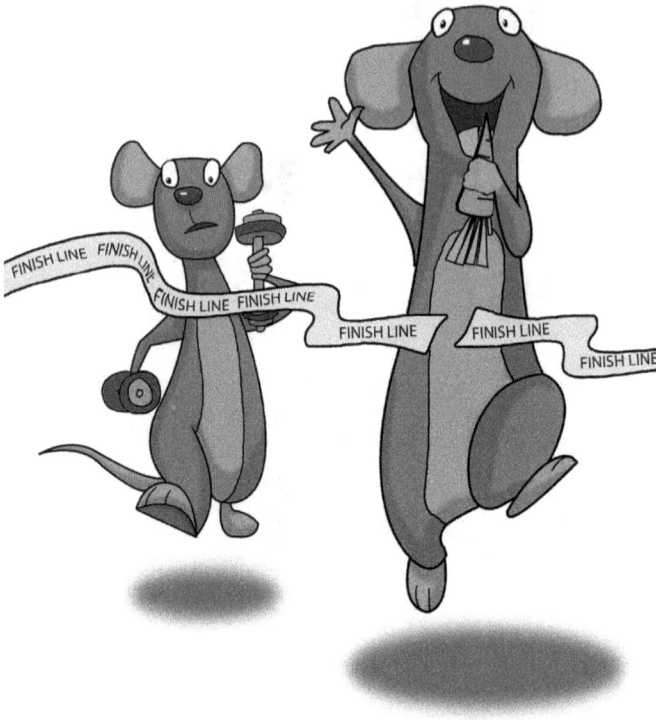

My patients often tell me that their physical activity is limited, for various reasons, resulting in more weight gain.

Let's examine this.

Famous weight loss coach Harper said that in his experience as a weight-loss coach, diet trumps exercise in weight loss. So let's examine this statement.

We will discuss exercise and its benefits in a later chapter.

This chapter will examine why diet, rather than exercise, is the most important thing for losing weight.

Scientists have been excited about this area of research lately, as they feel that the cure for the obesity may be found in the human gut. And be warned, there are other organisms in our body that control what we do by hacking our brain.

The bacteria-gut-brain axis

THE LINK BETWEEN BACTERIA IN THE GUT AND THE BRAIN

This chapter will shake to the core, your understanding of diets, calories, and eating habits.

So far we have been told that weight loss depends only on how many calories we eat and how many we spend. Nothing could be further from the truth. What we eat changes the type of bacteria and their ratio in our gut. So why does a change in the bacteria in our gut so important?

These are no ordinary bacteria; they have the ability to control our brain. It sounds terrifying, but it is the new emerging truth. And these bacteria may hold the key to weight loss.

Do you remember in the previous chapter on scientific research we talked about how gastric bypass surgery changes the bacteria in our gut? We will pick it up from there in this chapter

In this chapter will go through a series of completed scientific research on lab animals, including our beloved ratz. I have broken down what is quite complex research to make it easy to understand. What you will learn will change your thinking about food completely and blow your mind away.

I. The microbiome: The bacteria in our gut

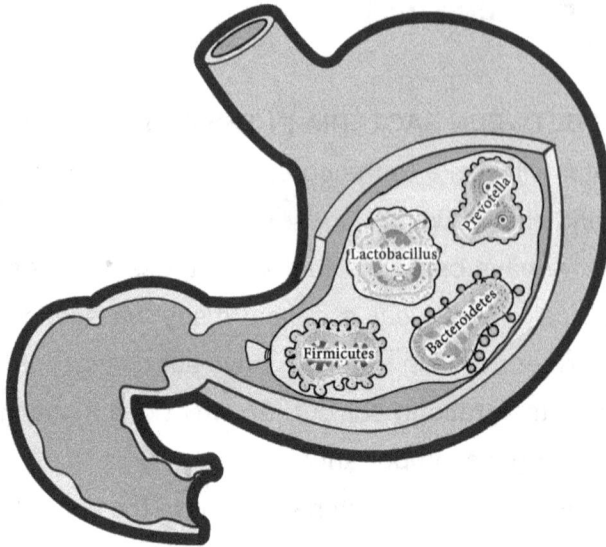

Let me introduce you to the gazillions of bacteria in the gut system. There are many different types and are present in different quantities in our gut. Together, they are called the **microbiome**.

Because individuals in different parts of the world, such as America or Asia, are exposed to different diets, the microbiome differs significantly in individuals around the world.

The composition of our gut bacteria — Microbiome — is established in the early years of life, in childhood. What you eat as a child, or what you feed your child, is very important. Over time, however, it can change, even in adulthood, due to many factors.

Major factors that affect the Microbiome include:

1. Microbiome passed from mother to child.
2. Your diet
3. Use of antibiotics
4. Stomach and other intestinal infections
5. Stress

The most abundant types of bacteria in the gut are *bacteroides, clostridium, fusobacterium, eubacterium, ruminococcus, peptococcus, peptostreptococcus,* and *bifidobacterium*. Escherichia and lactobacillus are also present in the gut, to a lesser extent.

All you need to remember is that there are two types of gut flora: Fat-Me-Not and Fat-Me-Yes compositions.

WHAT DO WE KNOW ABOUT THE GUT FLORA OR THE MICROBIOME?

We have 100 trillion microorganisms in our gut system. They are not living there for free. They help out in our body functions in the following ways:

1. Fermentation of undigested carbohydrates; when this function is disturbed, lactose intolerance, functional diarrhea, and abdominal bloating can result.
2. Short chain fatty acid absorption thus helping the integrity, immunity, and anti-inflammatory properties of the gut mucosa.
3. Metabolism of bile acid, antibiotics, and sterols (cholesterol, plant sterols): Through this task the gut flora help control cholesterol.

4. Production of vitamin K, vitamin B, and Biotin: Deficiency can result if the gut flora are altered in an undesirable pattern.

5. Modification of the immune system: Gut flora protects us from allergic reactions in a complex way. Too complex to discuss here in this book.

6. A normal gut flora limits the growth of harmful bacteria and preventing diseases and infections. For example when antibiotics destroy the good bacteria, the bad bacteria like C.difficile takes over and can cause severe infectious colitis.

7. They play a helpful role in treating inflammatory diseases such as Crohn disease, Ulcerative colitis, obesity, and metabolic diseases.

The bacteria in the microbiome can change in number and types as a result of several factors. For example, even a short course of mild antibiotics, such as azitromycin, can change the gut bacteria composition for more than six months. An acute change in diet, however, doesn't change the microbiome, so turning vegetarian for few months won't do you any good; it has to be a long-term change.

We will talk more about the microbiome later in this chapter when we discuss how these bacteria affect us. You may not be able to see them, but they can control your brain, and are thus able to control your appetite, your portions, your cravings, and even your stress levels.

II. The brain center for weight regulation: How the brain controls our weight

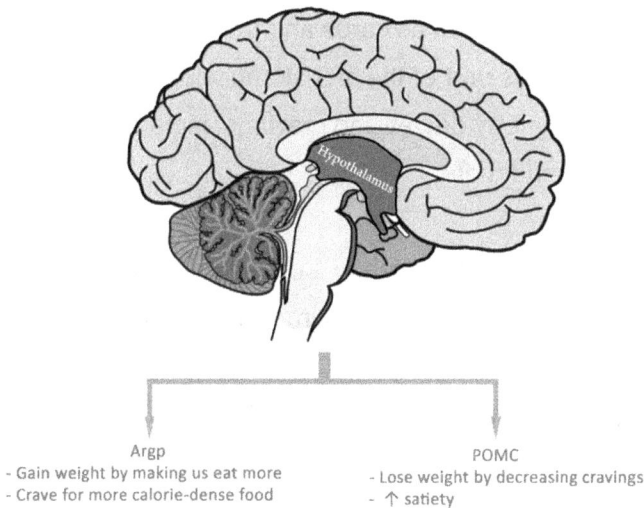

Argp
- Gain weight by making us eat more
- Crave for more calorie-dense food

POMC
- Lose weight by decreasing cravings
- ↑ satiety

One of the responsibilities of our brain is to make sure we are not losing weight beyond a certain limit. If we do, it threatens the body's survival. In the early days of human civilization, food was scarce, meaning that starvation was a real threat. As a result, the brain is geared to prevent us from losing weight, rather than helping us to lose weight.

However, now we have access to an abundant supply of food, including high-calorie processed foods, at least in the developed world. So such a tight guard on losing weight is no longer needed in humans. Unfortunately, the evolution of the brain lags behind in terms of developing the ability to prevent weight gain.

Weight is regulated in an area of the brain called the hypothalamus. In the hypothalamus, there is a nucleus (or a center) called the **arcuate nucleus**, or ARC.

This nucleus is divided into two parts:

1. **Argp:** is the part of the arcuate nucleus that helps increase weight by making us eat more and crave for more calorie-dense foods such as carbs and fat.

2. **POMC:** This part of the arcuate nucleus helps us lose weight by decreasing cravings, increasing satiety, and more.

This weight regulation center in the brain receives messages from the stomach from multiple sources, including:

1. The vagus nerve
2. Neuropeptides or gut hormones
3. Other pathways

In response to the messages it receives, the Argp or POMC part of the nucleus activates and sends back signals to control calorie intake, energy consumption, and more.

The balance between the activity of Argp and POMC decides our weight.

III. Gut hormones: Hormones secreted by the gut (stomach and intestines) that send messages to the brain

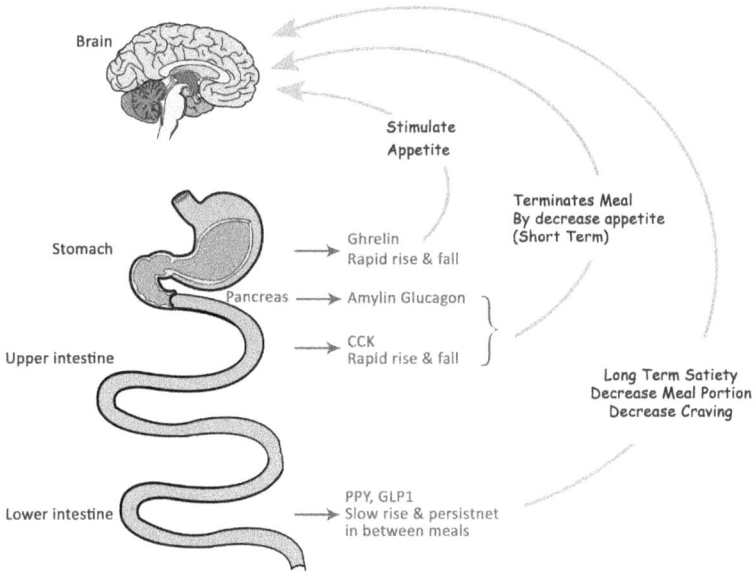

Hormones Secreted by Our Gut That Send Messages to Our Brain

The major neuropeptides or gut hormones secreted by the body include:

1. Ghrelin: Increases appetite
2. CCK: Decreases appetite and tells the brain to stop eating
3. PYY: Decreases appetite
4. GLP-1: Decreases appetite
5. OXM: Decreases appetite
6. Insulin: Decreases appetite
7. NPY: Increases food intake
8. Leptin: Opposite of ghrelin; counteracts NPY

The stomach secretes only ghrelin. The pancreas secretes insulin, while the intestines secrete the others.

Let's look at these gut messenger hormones in more depth.

GHRELIN
- Secreted by the stomach
- Increases stomach emptying and intestinal motility
- Propels food forward to make space for incoming food
- Forces the body to use glucose as energy source
- Makes us hungry

Ghrelin increases when it is time to eat. It makes us hungry. Too much ghrelin can cause overeating, and thus obesity.

CCK
- Secreted by the upper intestine
- Reduces sugar peak by slowing the movement of food in the system

Makes us feel full after a meal so we terminate the meal

PYY
- Secreted by the lower intestine
- Makes us feel full over a long period of time and thus controls how much we eat over several meals.

Burns fat as an energy source

GLP-1
- Secreted by the lower intestine
- Reduces sugar peak
- Increases insulin secretion

- Replenishes insulin stores
- Already used in diabetes treatment

GIP

- Causes insulin resistance and obesity
- If blocked, rats in the lab don't get obese
- Fat gets used as an energy source

IV. The Hacker Connection: How bacteria in the gut control the brain

The bacteria in the gut have the ability to send signals to the brain by manipulating the secretions of these gut hormones. They can alter signals going from the gut to the brain. The brain will act based on what it perceives the situation is in the gut, based on the signals from these hormones. There are other ways these bacteria can control our brain, but these are minor and outside the scope of this book. The bacteria send most of weight-related messages via the gut hormones to the brain. This results in a change in our eating behavior, metabolism, and use of carbs or fat as an energy source.

Research shows these bacteria can and do alter behavior, including eating behavior, which is important for weight gain and loss. We will discuss scientific research on all kinds of behavior that these bacteria can change so you can get an idea about the potential reach of these bacteria.

Research Study: Bacteria in the gut can alter sexual preference in fruit flies

Even though this research has nothing to do with weight loss I decided to include it to show how much control bacteria can exert on our behavior by hacking our nervous system.

In this study, one group of fruit flies was given a starch diet. The other group was given a malt diet. Interestingly, the starch-fed fruit flies mated with starch-fed fruit flies, while the malt-fed fruit flies mated only with other malt-fed fruit flies.

This mating preference lasted for more than thirty-seven generations. However, a simple course of antibiotics, destroying the bacteria in the fruit flies' guts, gets rid of this mating preference; the fruit flies start mating indiscreetly after receiving the antibiotics.

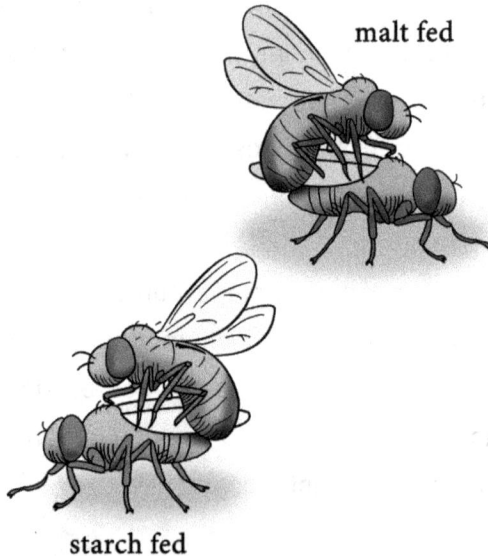

malt fed

starch fed

Bacteria in the gut can alter sexual preference in fruit flies

> *Bottom line: The gut bacteria has enormous amount of control on our brain. This study proves the bacteria can hack our nervous system.*

Research Study: Bacteria in the gut can improve stress levels, #1

In a Rat Maternal Separation Study, stress was induced in a baby rat by separating him from his mother. As a result, the baby rat wouldn't swim when put in water. This behavior got better once the baby rat was returned back to his mom.

They also found that the behavior got better if baby rats were given anti-depressants instead of being returned to their mothers.

When instead of doing any of the above, if gut bacteria called *B. infantis* were infused in the separated baby rat's gut, the baby rat got better; stress was resolved without needing to be reunited with Mom. Somehow, the new bacteria manipulated the signals going to the brain, making it feel better.

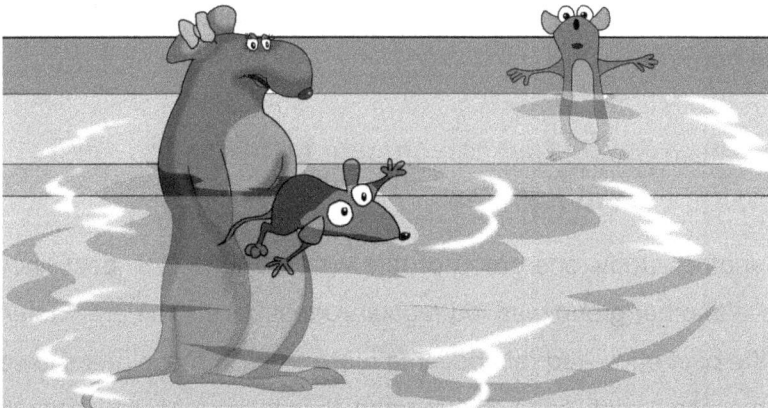

Good bacteria in the gut can improve stress level in rats

Research Study: Bacteria in the gut can improve stress levels, #2

In another study, extensive antibiotics made a group of rats germ-free in the gut. Their gut bacteria were completely wiped out by these antibiotics. They were noted to have exaggerated stress responses compared to those rats with normal microbiomes. If the microbiome or the gut bacteria from normal rats was added to the gut of these bacteria free rats, their stress response became normal.

If only a single gut bacteria named *E.coli* was added, the stress response became even more exaggerated in the germ-free rats. Then they tried to add *B. infantis* to the germ-free rats. The stress reaction normalized.

Research Study: Diet can change behavior and ability through the gut bacteria

In another study, one group of rats was fed 50% lean beef chow, while another group was fed regular rodent chow. The gut bacteria in the beef chow-fed rats became more diverse; these rats showed decreased anxiety and better memory than the rodent chow-fed rats.

This doesn't mean that eating beef will improve your memory and decrease your anxiety; we haven't yet proven this in humans. However, it does point to the fact that your diet can change the bacterial microbiome in your gut and thus change how you behave. So when Grandma said you are what you eat, she was right.

> *Bottom Line: Your diet can change bacteria in your gut. And the bacteria in your gut can change you.*

Research Study: Bacteria in the gut have the power to change blood pressure

In a study on rats, a bacteria called *Lactobacillus johnsonis* was injected into the duodenum, or upper intestine, of a group of rats. These rats showed improvement in their blood pressure as well as improvement in their stress hormone levels.

> *Bottom Line: Healthy eating, healthy bacteria in the gut may have many benefits.*

Research Study: Bacteria in the gut has the power to change weight

A group of rats was given a high-fat diet and their gut bacteria were studied with the intention of making them gain weight. The two major groups of microbiome (Fat-Me-Yes and Fat-Me-Not) of the microorganisms were studied.

With the fatty diet, the Fat-Me-Not bacteria waned and were replaced by increasing Fat-Me-Yes bacterial flora.

We want more Fat-Me-Not bacteria composition than Fat-Me-Yes bacteria in our gut.

The Fat-Me-Yes bacteria inflame the gut mucosa, making it angry-looking and causing it to store more calories and make us gain weight. Fat-Me-Yes bacteria also squeezes out more calories from the food you eat than Fat-Me-Not bacteria making you gain weight.

Research Study: Stool Transfer Study

Importing gut bateria via stool transplant

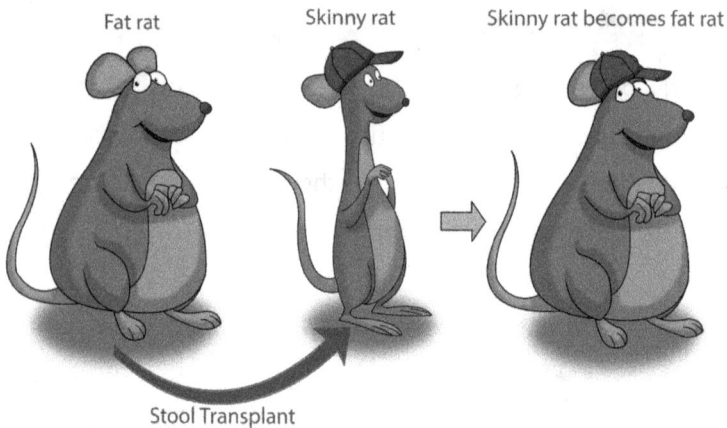

Fat rat   Skinny rat   Skinny rat becomes fat rat

Stool Transplant

The feces contains the sample of microbiome or gut bacteria we have. In another Mr. Ratz study, obese Mr. Ratz feces (which contains their microbiome sample) were injected into lean Mr. Ratz colon via an enema. Guess what happened, Lean Mr. Ratz become Obese Mr. Ratz. The importing of Fat-Me-Yes bacteria from obese rats made the lean rats gain weight.

After the Mr. Ratz findings, many human studies were done based on this hypothesis. The results are very convincing, suggesting that we can control our gut flora, and thus weight, through diet. Some researchers are hopeful that, if played correctly, this may turn out to be a medical bypass for weight loss.

POINTS

- Gut flora has a major effect on weight control.
- Diet changes the gut flora.

Diet trumps exercise

How do bacteria change our stress levels? It is likely that they do it by hacking the gut hormones and sending signals to the brain. Fat-Me-Not bacteria, the good bacteria in the gut are like an ethical hacker; they help us. Fat-Me-Yes bacteria are the Bad bacteria in the gut; their manipulation of gut hormones can affect our health and wellbeing in a negative way. Both work by hacking into our nervous system.

Scientific data suggests that we can change our gut bacteria composition with diet and therefore influence what these bacteria do to us. This is why, what and how we eat is so much more important than exercise. Eating properly for a few days or weeks will not help; you need to eat correctly forever. Only then will your gut bacteria be a healthy microbiome of Fat-Me-Not bacteria and provide you with beneficial results. This is the primary reason why people who eat healthy for a few weeks lose weight, only to gain the weight back once they stop. A short-term, quick fix diet will never work. Neither will a low-fat or low-carb diet. Balance is really important, as you have seen in all the research we discussed.

This is why we incorporated a balanced diet in SlimPlate System and emphasized that weight loss should be all about eating a balanced diet, not a limited diet. In addition, a non-limiting diet helps people to eat the right way for a long time without feeling deprived.

If we have an abundance of microbiome in Fat-Me-Yes predominance, these Fat-Me-Yes species of bacteria will hack into your nervous system and make you crave high-fat and high-processed diets so that they can survive. However, if we have Fat-Me-Not microbiome in us, it will still hack our nervous system but make us crave high-fiber, well-balanced diet, because that is the kind of diet these bacteria thrive on for its survival.

This brings us to a very important juncture. You are either trapped in a Fat-Me-Yes cycle or if you are lucky you are in a Fat-Me-Not cycle. If you crave junk food all the time, if you feel stressed, or if you gain weight without eat too much you are likely trapped in a Fat-Me-Yes cycle. You have to break free from the Fat-Me-Yes cycle and correct your diet to get into the Fat-Me-Not cycle. The only way to get out of vicious Fat-Me-Yes cycle is to switch your diet to healthy well-balanced and well portioned diet. But the good news is that once you are out of the Fat-Me-Yes cycle and well in to the Fat-Me-Not cycle maintaining your weight will be a lot easier, your cravings will go down, you will automatically be looking for healthier food and you will feel less stressed. Now study the two cycles in the picture very carefully as this is where you have to make the switch for losing weight and keep it off. Later we will discuss how to make this switch in detail.

This amazing discovery of how the bacteria in our body control us reminds me of puzzling medical stories I have experienced in the past.

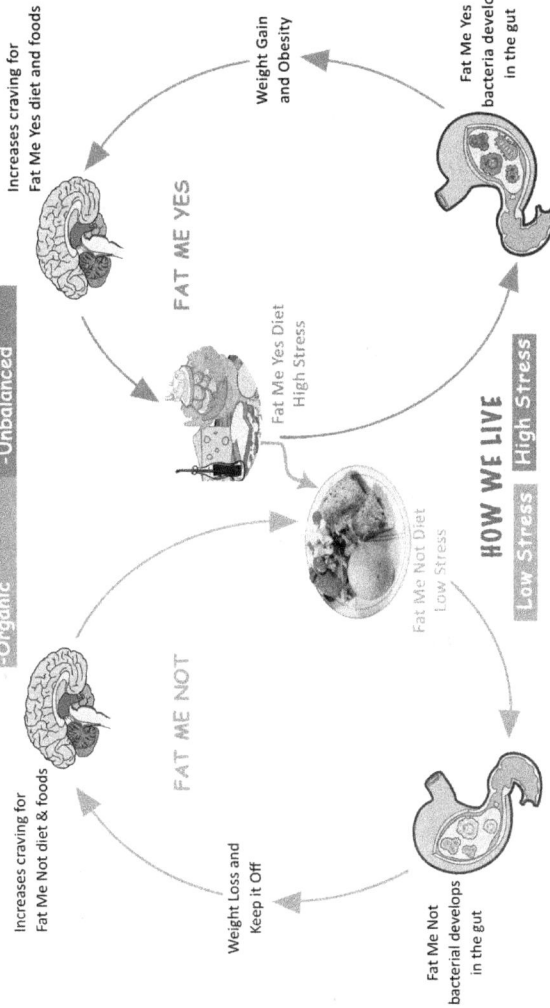

HOW WE EAT

- Balanced
- Portion-Controlled
- High Fiber
- Organic

- Deprived Diet
- High Fat Diet
- Processed food
- Unbalanced

FAT ME YES CYCLE

Increases craving for Fat Me Yes diet and foods

FAT ME YES

Weight Gain and Obesity

Fat Me Yes bacteria develops in the gut

Fat Me Yes Diet
High Stress

HOW WE LIVE Low Stress High Stress

What does Fat-Me-Yes Bacteria Do?
- Increase inflammation
- Squeeze more calories out and also causes gas
- Hack the body gut to release Fat-Me-Yes gut hormones

FAT ME NOT CYCLE

Increases craving for Fat Me Not diet & foods

FAT ME NOT

Weight Loss and Keep it Off

Fat Me Not bacterial develops in the gut

Fat Me Not Diet
Low Stress

What does Fat-Me-Not Bacteria Do?
- Decrease inflammation
- Does not squeeze too many calories from food we eat
- Hack the body gut to release Fat-Not gut hormones

Fat-me-not and Fat-me-yes cycles

Chapter 8: Why Diet Trumps Exercise? 209

MARGARET

Margaret was a patient of mine early on in my weight-loss practice; she weighed 256 pounds. I saw her frequently for multiple sicknesses; she'd be in my clinic every two weeks. She had been like this for many years, and often changed doctors as she felt she wasn't treated well enough or that she was unable to get appointments easily enough whenever she got sick.

Margaret came to see me for frequent episodes of oral thrush (fungal infections), frequent diarrhea, or upper respiratory and sinus infection.

She didn't smoke. We went through with environmental allergy testing, food allergy testing, and gluten sensitivity testing, as well as a stool work up, including bacteria, cultures, yeast culturing, and every other possible and available test.

At the time, I didn't know that obesity might be responsible for all of her problems.

One day, her only son was getting married; Margaret wanted to lose weight for the wedding. She came in, excited, and told me that she needed my help to lose weight, the same way I'd been helping her with her illnesses, so that she could get ready for her son's wedding.

She signed up for my weight-loss clinic; she was one of my earliest weight-loss patients.

That time we did not have the SlimPlate System but were using in home portion control diet plan. She went through with then in-house portion control diet plan weight loss program and lost thirty-six pounds before her son's wedding. She was ready to face her friends and family to show off her new look.

The first time I saw her back in the medical clinic was six months after her son's wedding. She had stayed leaner, and I was surprised that she hadn't come back for the little illnesses as she had done before.

I asked her how her stomach, sinus, and oral thrush were feeling.

She said that she felt better and that none of her previous illnesses had returned, and wanted to know if the last round of antibiotics had killed everything off.

I was sure that the last antibiotic, was no different from the many other she had been prescribed and therefore couldn't be curing all of her little illnesses. That left me with an unanswered puzzle.

Now, looking back, I know that because of her weight loss, she was able to get rid of all of her illnesses. If we could go back in time and check to compare her gut flora before and after, we would definitely see a change from Fat-Me-Yes to Fat-Me-Not. This explains how her frequent inflammation, unexplained abdominal pain, diarrhea, hypersensitivities to food, and low immunity with frequent infections for which she frequently visited the doctor during her early decades, completely resolved. In actuality, many antibiotics that were being used on her further changed her gut flora in an undesirable way and she was stuck in the Fat-Me-Yes cycle.

WHAT CAN CHANGE THE COMPOSITION OF OUR GUT FLORA?

1. *Composition of the diet can change the gut flora, for better or worse*

   Change for the worse: Fat-Me-Yes bacteria

   a) High-fat/low-carb diet

   b) High-carb/low-fat diet

Change for the better: Fat-Me-Not bacteria

a) Balanced diet with high protein

b) High-fiber diet

Your diet should be high in both fiber and protein. Eat whole grains and leave refined or processed versions of bread and other carbs out of your diet.

Don't confuse wholegrain with wheat, however; wheat is the name of a grain. As long as the bread or carb is 100% wholegrain, it doesn't matter if it's made of wheat, rye, oats, barley, or any other grains. Flour should be ground from the entire grain. Often the outer shell of grains are polished and refined, and are then made into refined flour. Flour made from whole grains is a much better choice than polished, refined flour.

2. *Many antibiotics can change the composition of the gut flora*

In the United States, antibiotic use is increasing. This is one of the reasons that we're obese as a country.

We use antibiotics commonly, many a times when it is not needed. The meat we eat is also from animals treated with antibiotics for sickness and growth.

Every day, we're exposed to antibiotics, either through prescriptions or through the food we ingest.

Antibiotics, either through a chronic low dose ingested through food or the antibiotics taken for our illnesses, can alter the natural gut flora to Fat-Me-Yes composition.

Buy organic products; wild seafood, for instance, in preference to farm-raised ones.

Don't use antibiotics easily. Most seasonal infections are viral and don't require antibiotics. Ask your doctor not to prescribe you antibiotics unless absolutely necessary.

Amoxicillin is a safer antibiotic for our gut flora, but your doctor will select the antibiotics that are best suited to treating any infections that you might have.

3. *Probiotics*

Probiotics are microorganisms (synthetic gut flora) that are commonly used and may alter the gut flora. Many researchers work in this area, specifically looking at the kinds of probiotic microorganisms that will help with specific diseases.

Probiotics can be used for many therapeutic uses for various diseases, including antibiotic-induced diarrhea, vaginosis (vaginal infection), helicobacter pylori infection, lactose intolerance, inflammatory bowel disease, and a few others. Composition can vary, especially with human diet and overall health. Currently there is no definite use of probiotics for obesity.

4. *Prebiotics*

Prebiotics are non-digestible fibers that come from food; they pass through the stomach to the large intestine and make changes in the microbiome in favor of human wellbeing and health.

High-fiber diets are beneficial for the wellbeing and health of humans; and can be found in beans, raw wheat, raw oats, barley, garlic, leeks, onions, asparagus, Jerusalem artichokes, and chicory root.

5. *Weight loss*

   The Fat-Me-Not microorganism helps us to lose weight. Once you're lean, Fat-Me-Not microorganisms become abundant in the body.

   We have to start somewhere to get the Fat-Me-Not micro-organisms into the gut. A Fat-Me-Not diet will get you into a Fat-Me-Not cycle. This is why starting out with the right diet is crucial to losing weight. The rest will automatically follow. Body weight is controlled by Fat-Me-Not and Fat-Me-Yes gut flora via gut hormones that send signals to the brain. The brain then determines appetite, craving, energy expenditure, and energy storage according to the signal that has been sent.

   So find out if you are stuck in Fat-Me-Yes cycle and if you are, it is time to switch your diet to enter the Fat-Me-Not cycle.

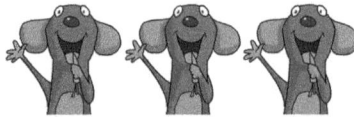

Chapter 9

What Prevents Us From Losing Weight?

And How to Fix it

Why should I lose weight?

1. I want to be able to cross my legs.
2. I want to be able to fit in restaurant booths.
3. I want to be able to bend down.
4. I want to be able to reach my back.
5. I want to be able to reach my legs and tie my shoes.
6. I want to be able to do chores as others do without needing help.
7. I want to be able to get up easily and reach things.
8. I want to feel comfortable in the chairs I sit in.
9. I want to feel comfortable and confident in myself and what others will think of me.
10. I want to be able to go through entrances and exits without being embarrassed.
11. I want my body to feel light.
12. I want to be able to go anywhere without restriction.
13. I want to play with my kids.
14. I want to be healthy.
15. I want to take fewer medications for my medical problems.
16. I want to relieve my aching joints.
17. I want to relieve my foot pain.
18. I want to relieve my sleep apnea.
19. I want to improve my blood pressure, cholesterol, and blood sugar.
20. I want to get out of the cycle of taking more medications and gaining more weight.
21. I want to feel better about my life, my future, my health, and myself.

Whatever your reason is the time to lose weight is now.

How to deal with the barriers of losing weight

TIME

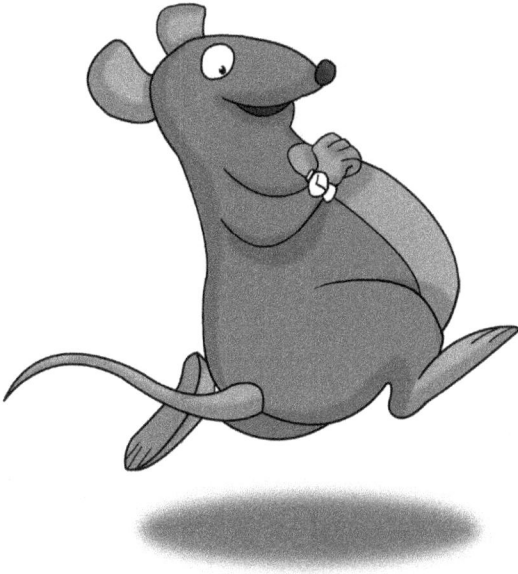

Life is always busy with tasks and schedules. We have to prioritize; losing weight has to be at the top of the list. It is a matter of your health and without health you have nothing.

Keep your goals small in the beginning and ask for support. Tell your family that you are planning to lose seven pounds in one month and ask for help and support to keep your goal in check.

MONEY

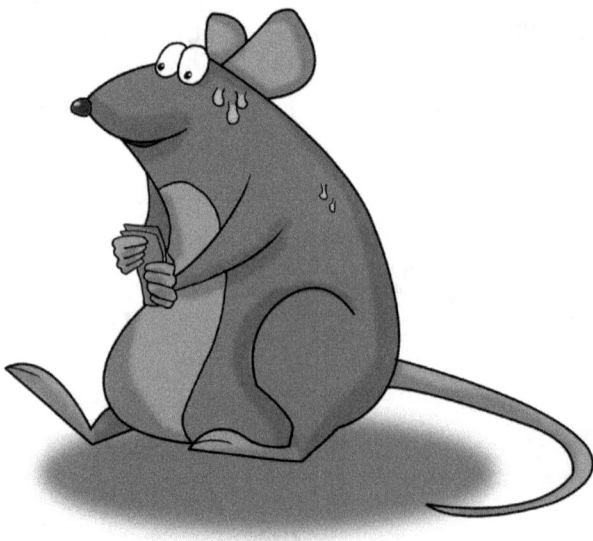

Losing weight can come with some costs, whether it's joining a program, buying equipment, SlimPlate System, and/ or purchasing healthier grocery.

Again, you need to prioritize. Cut back on buying non-essential items but don't cut back on your weight-reduction efforts. Delaying your weight management is more costly in the long run. As you lose weight, you will begin to realize that you can cut back on medications, doctor's visits, sick days and loss of income etc., and thus save a lot more money; more than you put in initially.

I see a lot of patients in consultation who don't pursue weight loss, nor do they stop smoking, because insurance companies won't pay for smoking cessation medications and weight-loss plans. As a result, they continue to spend money on cigarettes and do not change their unhealthy habits.

Here, the key is to lose weight and adopt healthy habits for your own health. It would be nice to have wellness coverage, but if you don't have that coverage you should have an alternative plan in place. This may include working extra shifts to cover the cost of treatment, or cutting back on other non-essential buys. Remember, by losing weight and ceasing smoking, you'll actually save a lot more money.

KNOWLEDGE

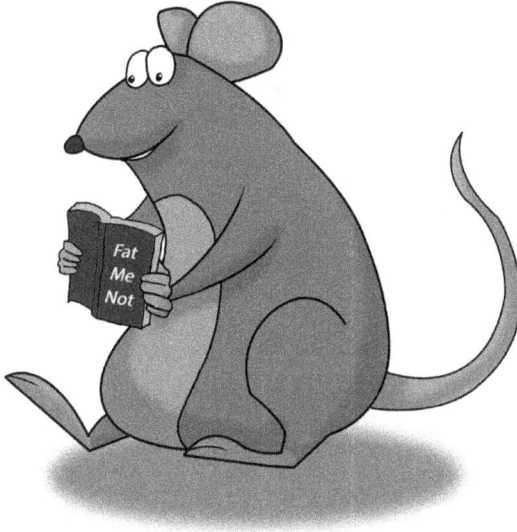

Knowledge is power. Look for true facts and correct information about weight loss and weight loss programs. Don't rely on information that you receive from advertisements. Advertisements mainly serve to sell merchandise.

Don't look for a quick fix. There is no quick and easy way of losing weight. You have to go through with the diet, exercise, and adopting of the right habits and medications (diet pills) if you can safely take them. We have made SlimPlate System to make it easier for our patients to lose weight. You can also get one for yourself from www.slimplatesystem.com.

DETERMINATION

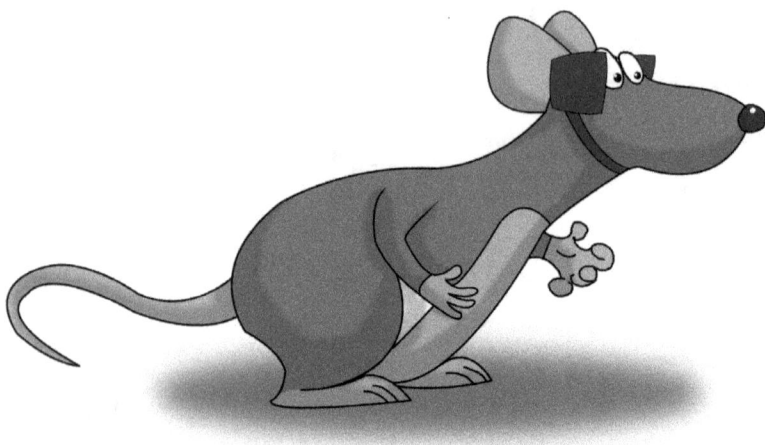

Once you decide to lose weight, it's important to keep the goal alive until you achieve it. Don't lose sight of the goal. There will be festivals, parties, life stresses, plans that fail, difficulties, and all kinds of excuses, whether reasonable or not. You must keep your eyes on the goal and continue with your efforts.

Get support from friends and family. Think and reward yourself with non-food item for your achievements. If you have shortcomings, correct them positively.

I have said it many times: it is easy to lose weight, so be encouraged.

After losing weight, we owe it to ourselves to maintain the lost weight. This goal should accompany your weight-loss plan from day one.

It is fun to lose weight. Think of all the good things that are going to come your way. You will be in less pain, will be able to engage in more activity, you will look nicer and be happier... Everything that you can imagine that's good in life will come with weight loss.

I see people come back to see me after losing weight; thrilled and happy, some even dance. No one comes back upset about having lost weight.

Losing weight is fun and easy, but many people hate to even attempt losing weight because they think it is hard or it has to be hard, and are doubtful that it will work. It seems like trying to lose weight will only result in suffering.

The main reason I wrote this book was to revolutionize what we think about weight loss. New research shows it is a lot easier to lose weight than we thought before.

In the past, the weight loss industry has made you think:

1. *Losing weight is an emotional and physical restraint and pain.*

    This is not the case. You can eat what you got used to eating growing up, and you can still lose weight.

    You don't need to feel deprived or crave anything, because you can eat everything that you like. No low carb or low fat or no fad diets anymore.

2. *Losing weight means you must suffer and go through hardships.*

    Since 2007, I've been trouble-shooting the challenges my weight-loss patients encounter. I have yet to see someone give up because it's too hard to follow. My patients never felt it was hard. Many never realized they were on a diet plan.

    I don't believe that you need to go out of your way to lose weight. Efforts made to lose weight should only go your way. Unlearn the idea that weight loss has to be hard.

3. *Will it work, or will it disappoint me?*

    It's good to be skeptical when thinking about which weight-loss technique is the best option for you to achieve long-term results.

    Generally, you should choose a weight-loss program that meets three major criteria:
    a) It should be easy.
    b) You can eat real food.
    c) It trains good habits for long-term weight-loss.

    Before you begin, ask yourself if the diet plan will let you eat real food; if you can keep it up for life; and if you can form good habits after a few months that will be easy to maintain for the rest of your life. If yes to all three, that is the diet plan for you.

    Can you buy special protein or frozen foods for life?

Can you count and measure everything you eat for life?

Can you continue buying supplements, pills, and powders for life?

Can you keep getting shots for life?

Can you keep eating protein bars and drinks for life?

Can you keep juicing for life?

Can you eat raw food for life?

The answer is all of the above cannot be sustained for rest of your life. Some of these may work, but the effects won't last and will cause disappointment by rebound weight gain.

CHERYL

Cheryl was young and healthy and came to see me for a medical follow up. When I first entered the room, I thought she was a new patient; she had lost fifty pounds in five months, and I barely recognized her.

She was thrilled by her new look.

You all know by now that I'm really passionate about Fat-Me-Not stuff.

I understand my patients' challenges and share them. Obesity and its treatment has rooted in me as a passion and obsession to treat. I am always open to learning new things that will work so I can help others. Whenever something new comes up in the weight loss industry, I am immediately on it and checking it out. I know that I will get a ton of questions from my patients, and I want to know how I can best utilize the new techniques to help my patients, provided that the underlying science is sound.

Cheryl told me that she'd seen an old high school friend at church; the girl was lean and had lost a lot of weight, so Cheryl asked for her secret. It turns out that her friend had recently broken up with her boyfriend, and to get him back she wanted to look good. So she joined a HCG clinic, and used the HCG shot and the accompanying diet to lose weight.

Cheryl went to her friend's HCG clinic. She told me she didn't want to do the calorie counting, so she chose to do the protein diet with HCG shot.

Cheryl lost fifty pounds in five months.

All of my awe and curiosity disappeared and I went quiet. I couldn't be happy for her, as I knew what would happen in the next few months.

I knew it because I had seen it happen many times with my patients, time and again. By the time my patients come to me, they have failed numerous times at losing weight.

Cheryl told me that she had lost this weight and that she was now going to be put on a maintenance phase in which she would be reintroducing carbs. She was looking forward to that maintenance phase; she felt she had accomplished something significant by losing fifty pounds.

I didn't want to be the one to break the news that the weight loss would be temporary and that she would gain it back. At the same time, I was her doctor and it was my job to guide her correctly.

I asked her how her friend was doing. Cheryl said that her friend had gained back all of her weight, but that she is back with her boyfriend and wasn't following the plan anymore.

She didn't notice my silence.

She excitedly showed me that all of her subcutaneous fat had gone away.

I saw that all of her skin was loose and stretchy; we could pull it out a few inches.

When someone loses so much weight, it seems so real, especially when you can see where the fat's dropped away under the skin. I could see it with my own eyes, but that the same time I also knew that all that weight would come back.

This is how you gain the weight back after stopping your weight loss efforts.

After the pounds drop off, the balance of the body mechanism is altered, as is the gut hormones. Remember, there are two different pathways of gut-brain signaling; one is Fat-Me-Yes and the other is Fat-Me-Not. If a body maintains a stable weight, the balance between them is stable. As we lose weight, the balance between them changes.

The body has a survival instinct that recognizes (intentional) dieting and the effect of weight loss. It recreates and reverses the weight loss effect by shifting the balance between Fat-Me-Not and Fat-Me-Yes. In this post-dieting and active weight-loss phase, the body increases the Fat-Me-Not and decreases the Fat-Me-Yes hormones. But because the weight loss effort is temporary and cannot be sustained here, as the diet changes back, the gut bacteria and hormones return to Fat-Me-Yes. And when the Fat-Me-Yes bacteria come back the second time they act with vengeance. Both your body and bacteria, in tandem, causing Fat-Me-Yes hormone surge, demanding more of the unhealthy food, driving your cravings through the roof. The final result? Rebound weight gain; way more than before.

When we are overwhelmed and dragged down by Fat-Me-Yes hormones, our willpower can't resist for long. Rebound weight gain is inevitable.

Just as a side-note, scientists are looking at this Fat-Me-Yes hormone surge. There are a few hormones related actions, such as promoting Leptin and reducing Grehlin, are being studied for long-term weight management. These hormones may become treatment options for losing weight in the near future. There are also other things we can do to resist the Fat-Me-Yes hormone surge; I will discuss them in the Fat-Me-Not success plan.

POINTS

- Don't do weight loss for few months, do it for a lifetime.
- Make sure the weight loss plan meets the three criteria
- Don't let your body feel that you're going far away from your normal self in an attempt to lose weight. The further you go from your normal self, the easier it will be for the weight to return. The more magical or drastic it seems, the more difficult it is to avoid regaining weight.

MICHELLE

Michelle was a famous, rich entrepreneur who wanted to improve her looks. She weighed twenty-five pounds more than what she wanted.

Michelle saw me in my weight-loss clinic; she was losing three to six pounds per month. As an entrepreneur, she carried a lot of tension as a result of pressure from her work. She always came in with a great deal of stress.

Her role meant that she was on TV and in front of the media, so she really worried about her looks. At about five feet in height, she said that the TV cameras could pick up even a small weight change.

Stress and lack of time hindered her weight-loss progress. She couldn't eat as regularly as she wanted to and she was always red in the face, with clenched teeth and soft but cursing outbursts.

She came in and talked about her business partners, her employees, her competitors, and all of her stress. Most of our session was to practice her pulling herself out of her own body so she could watch as a third party. This let her think and see how little her problems were, and to consider how easy it would be to solve her little problems. I basically became her psychiatrist.

I let her see that what she thought were huge problems were actually small challenges; the goal was for her to learn to tackle her problems without suffering from large amounts of stress.

One day, Michelle came in and confessed that she had gone to a spa and she had had a procedure done to melt the fat away from her belly.

She swore that she saw the fat coming out of her urine like sediment; she thought she was losing fat. The more she drank water, the more she saw fat in her urine, and she felt that her belly fat was shedding.

I always believe in my patients, and I didn't think she wasn't telling the truth.

My question was how this could be possible in the human body. I was curious how fat could get to the kidneys in order to be released through the urine.

Fat, that was lost in that way was not visceral, but subcutaneous fat. Visceral fat is the bad kind that puts the body in inflammatory mode and causes various diseases.

Visceral fat is commonly seen inside the peritoneal cavity; it mixes with and infiltrates the intra-abdominal organs such as the liver, pancreas, gut, and spleen.

Subcutaneous fat is the layer of fat underneath the skin all over the body. Wherever there is loose space, fat tends to accumulate, so that's why we see love handles, subcutaneous belly bulges, and fat around the hip, buttock, and breast tissues. Usually subcutaneous fat intermingles with cutaneous collagen and fibrous tissues, but too much can disturb the architectural layer of subcutaneous fat and make fat hang down from the belly.

There are multiple ways to remove subcutaneous fat, including low-level laser, radiofrequency, cryo-lipolysis, high intensity focused ultrasound, and liposuction.

Body contouring surgery is another procedure to take out subcutaneous fat.

Procedures such as those mentioned above destroy the fat at the treatment spot of the subcutaneous area, like the blemishes on the face skin are destroyed. Liposuction dissolves the fat in the area and is taken out with suction.

But it is impossible for the melted fat to be discarded through the kidney system or for weight to be lost in that way. The kidneys function to save nutrients to the body; they must sieve all protein, glucose, and fat and keep them inside the circulatory system. Normally, the kidney will not excrete protein, fat, or sugar.

If the kidney is excreting these fat lobules like she said, it is a sick kidney.

Therefore, it isn't possible for fat to be excreted through the kidneys to such an extent that any weight can be lost. Fat that is taken out or destroyed by the above procedures can be done on subcutaneous fat and are more for body contouring rather than weight loss. These techniques are used for the spot destruction of a few pounds of fat on the surface.

Only very small particles can come out through urine; there is no way we can lose fat in sufficient amounts to claim weight loss.

Michelle spent several hundreds of dollars for that technique in the hopes that she would lose weight.

Every day, I feel pain at how my patients desperately try to get a few pounds off and cling to any promising technique they see in the market.

I explained to Michelle that this method was not a viable one for losing weight, especially visceral fat. I told her that if she wanted to have a perfectly trimmed body, she could pursue laser or liposuction. But she need to realize that Laser liposuction is for surface/subcutaneous fat; it isn't for weight loss.

Michelle weighed 130 pounds. She was not as chunky as she thought. But she wanted her body as a perfect as a sculpture. She might have had a maximum of three pounds in her belly bulge and one pound in each side of her love handles. If she wanted to have liposuction to remove that fat, she could do so.

There is nothing wrong with liposuction; even I want a perfect, toned body. Any time a bulge appears, I squeeze it and I wish it would go away. These little bulges sometimes make me more motivated to be active and watchful of what and when I eat.

But we need to be realistic. When you carry fifty extra pounds, you can't hope that these fat-melting techniques will melt away all of your fat. That is impossible.

As for Michelle seeing sediments in her urine — she may not have noticed before, but you can normally see certain sediments in your urine, especially during the menstrual period or mid-cycle, as well as during some other situations like kidney stones and metabolic disorders.

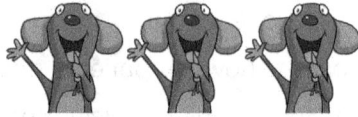

Chapter 10

Our SlimPlate System Journey

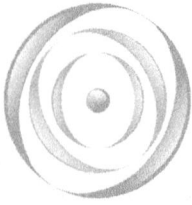

SLIMPLATE®
S Y S T E M
Weight Loss in a Box™

This chapter focuses on the how I developed the Fat-Me-Not success plan. I didn't draw up this plan overnight. I first had to understand obesity and then I had to understand its impact on people.

Since 2007, I have travelled many routes to help my obese patients. I have tried several meal replacements on the market, low-carb diets, low-calorie diets, and many kinds of medications. I have observed and followed many patients in their attempts to lose weight with different plans.

I now practice based on the Fat-Me-Not success plan. It has worked for my patients for the longest time in most effective way. Here is the history of how it all came together.

Dr. Nwe's diet in 2007

The diet I used to prescribe in 2007 was the easiest one to develop: working out how patients would measure food in their hands.

I taught patients to put two hands on their plate; one palm is the meat or protein. The top part of the hand is starch, while the second hand is vegetables.

I had some different ideas about how to pair foods in the plates. I developed snack lists, sweets lists, and breakfast lists so my patients could jump start on the plan.

We sat down and planned the meal plan per their choices.

At that time, I also used the plan in conjunction with meal replacement shakes and bars.

Often, patients came back within a few months and had already distorted their hand portions. They mixed things up with their own prior knowledge.

Then we decided to make the weight loss diet plan more structured. And step it up to the next level.

Portion plates 2008

A set of plates, bowls, cups, and a sandwich belt were drawn on paper, designed the way we like to eat.

My patients would leave the clinic with a set of paper plates, bowls, and cups as well as a sandwich belt and other bakery belt.

For any carbohydrate items, such as breakfast items, I gave patients the strips of paper (like a belt around a sandwich), allowing them to measure and cut out the extra portion

I went to kitchenware stores to get ideas and to get portion molds for different things people eat. Then I realized that people eat many different things. So I grouped them according to similarities of make and calories.

I went to many grocery stores to check calories and ingredients and figured out the desired amount that I wanted my patients to eat. There are tons of varieties of food to eat in this world.

Again, I came back and taught my patients what was out there and what we would do. But remember, even measuring with your own hands for a few major food groups was complicated for the majority of patients.

I realized that people shouldn't be learning many new things when trying to lose weight. If it's inconvenient for daily use, people won't follow it for long. They'll do it one day, maybe a week, but they won't keep it up for long.

We can't lose weight in a single week.

Remember, my focus from the very beginning was not for my patients to lose 30-40 pounds. My focus was on how they were going to continuously lose weight and keep the weight off forever. That has always been my focus and still is.

I had to constantly define where and when and why people lost their desire to continue to lose weight. I wanted to fix that part of the weight loss.

That was how SlimPlate System was born.

SlimPlate System was born in 2009

I was getting good at designing plates, bowls, and belts for different foods. I made them for men and women as well as multiple bowls for different food items.

One day I had a brainstorm session with my co-inventor, Dr. Grewal. We had a single objective to create a weight loss program that would be easy for patients to use, as well as successful, and that would encourage them to continue to lose weight.

Dr. Grewal, who is one of the most intuitive and innovative men that I have ever met, was a tremendous asset in developing a simple to use portion control system which portions everything under the sun. This way patient won't have to learn the whole science of nutrition to get out of Fat-Me-Yes cycle and enter the Fat-Me-Not cycle. We had many long discussions, arguments, and disagreements throughout putting together what now is the popular SlimPlate System.

Finally we scrapped everything extra and pared the system down to the minimum we needed for daily use.

To design it we had to meet all our objectives:
1. It should be easy to use
2. It should be good habit-forming
3. Nothing much to learn about nutrition
4. Durable
5. Intuitive
6. Aesthetically pleasing
7. Universal
8. Adaptable
9. One time cost – should not require people to spend money every month.
10. Efficacious

We designed a four-step systematic portion control weight-loss program, while combining the men and women plates into one and making it simple to use. Unless you're a professionally trained athlete, most people's calorie requirements aren't much different.

Over time, I have reviewed thousands of data point analysis of our patients' bodies, including basal metabolic rate, fat percent, lean mass percent, and water percent.

What I discovered from that data was most women require approximately 1500 calories daily and that men need approximately 1800 calories per day. It does not vary much.

Based on that, we made an easy-to-use system by making two different circles; the outer circle was for men and the inner circle was for women, indicating one meal of the day.

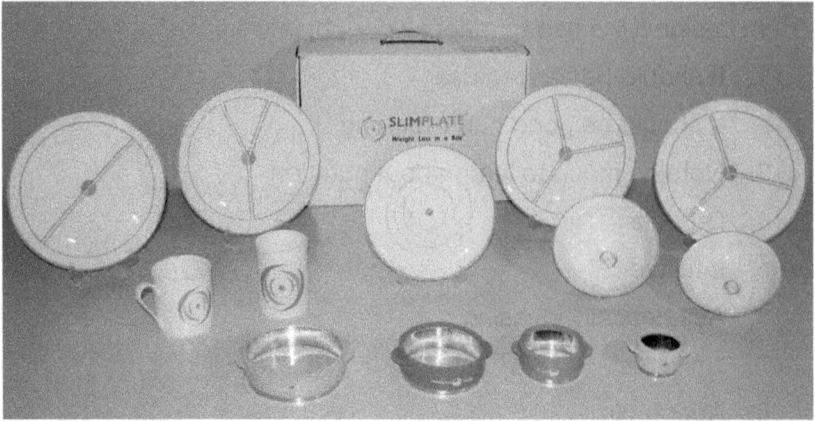

Complete SlimPlate System

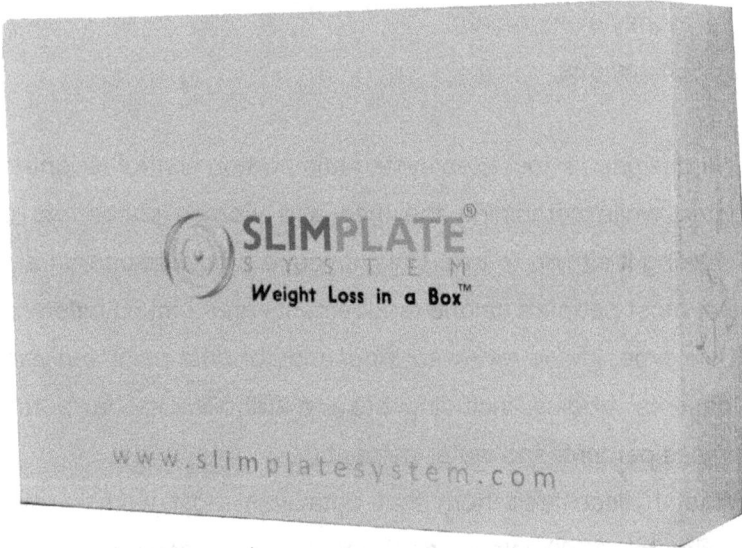

Weight Loss in a Box

Efficacy, sustainability, and long-term maintenance in 2012

We collected data on SlimPlate users from 2009 until 2011. We found that

1. Every SlimPlate System user lost weight.
2. The average weight loss was 14-22 pounds in the first three months.
3. The weight loss was sustainable beyond two years.
4. Average initial weight was 223 pounds.
5. Average age was 52 years old.

We were thrilled with the results. We presented the research at the American Society of Bariatric Physicians' annual meeting in 2012 in Orlando, Florida. Other physicians overwhelmingly supported us. The concept of the step portion control weight loss was widely perceived as positive by fellow physicians.

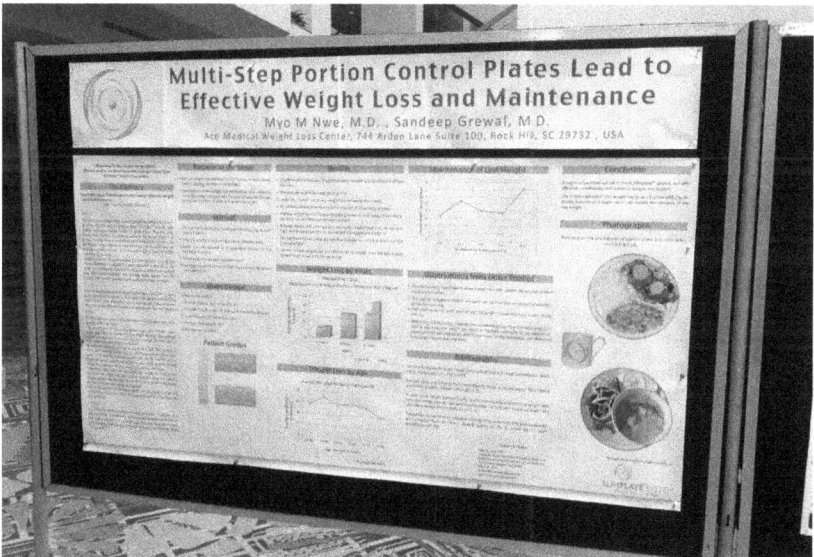

SlimPlate System results

Getting the SlimPlate System made

Initially we used disposable plates and cups. But disposable plates made people think they were in temporary mode; we wanted this to be a lifestyle change.

That led us to manufacture the SlimPlate System in fine bone china.

I selected a few companies and visited them. Then we chose one company based on its quality and durability. We visited their chemical labs and the entire factory to ensure safety and quality. SlimPlate System is not made with bone remains from animals, unlike other bone china plates. We wanted to make sure that vegetarians and non-meat-eaters didn't have to worry about eating on our high-quality bone china. SlimPlate is made with special LaLuna technology, which doesn't include actual animal bone. It is amazing how much I had to learn about manufacturing as a physician.

After selection, our design team and their manager worked on the prototype for several months before beginning product development.

First container, beginning of 2013

When the SlimPlate system arrived to our storage facility and then arrived to our office, we were incredibly excited.

The manufacturing was just perfect.

Our patients were excited to see it in beautiful bone china plates. Many of them got it in the first weeks and gave us lots of positive feedback.

One of them asked if she could imprint her name on it. She took pride in having a nice plate for herself.

Most of them said they could eat on these plates forever and continue to lose weight. We could see they enjoyed eating on SlimPlates.

That is what we intended to do. This is a lifestyle. This will be your dinnerware set. This will last forever.

Opening up our weight loss program to the world

Initially we had planned to make SlimPlate System available to our weight loss clinic patients only. But soon we decided give access to SlimPlate System to people all over the United States. Today you can also order a set for yourself at *www.slimplatesystem.com*. My weight loss coaches follow up with users nationally to ensure they continue to use the system and lose weight.

I insist on feedback from my coaches who are in touch with users everywhere. One day, I was told that a woman hadn't opened her set yet, though she'd had it for a week.

I take my patients' weight loss journey very personally.

In our clinic, my patients leave excited to open their SlimPlate System; they immediately download the SlimPlate App and are ready to start their weight loss journey.

So that feedback actually made me think.

How do I reach people far away from my office to help them lose weight? I know that we help so many people lose weight, not because of any magic, but because we almost hold our patients' hands, walking alongside them in their journey. It's important that we're in this weight-loss journey together.

How can we hold hands across the country?

Then we decided to start the SlimPlate Online Weight-Loss Program, in time for New Year 2014.

SlimPlate Online Weight Loss Program

In 2014 we launched our online weight-loss program. Our mission is to extend our imaginary helping hands to wrap around the nation and lose weight together.

We took the practical approach of
1. How to reset the metabolism
2. How to maximize fat-burning
3. How to eat in the correct portions for every food
4. How to eat correctly while eating out
5. How to handle stress and not to let your waistline grow
6. How to travel, party, and handle temptation
7. How to ward off food craving, binging, and addiction
8. How to improve physical activity, exercise, and be energetic

This is a four-month monthly program; people around the nation can participate from the convenience of their homes. Registration for this program is very easy and free; all you need is an email address and you'll be ready to embark on a weight-loss program with thousands of people around the nation.

Website: http://www.slimplatesystem.com/register

Understanding Systematic Portion Control

The word Portion control is very commonly used but is also misunderstood. Portion control is essentially going from a larger portion to a smaller portion, and it does help improve behavioral overeating. This isn't the same, however, as **systematic portion control**, which leads to weight loss.

WHAT IS A SYSTEMATIC PORTION CONTROL WEIGHT LOSS SYSTEM?

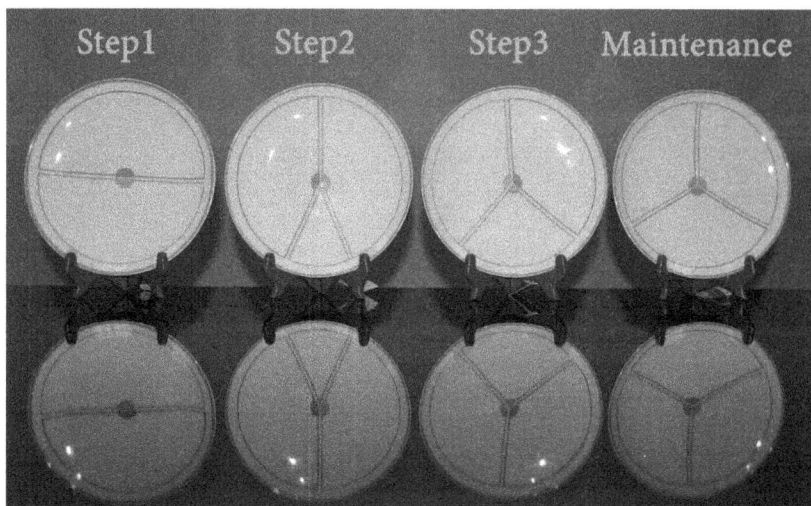

In systematic portion control we take the users through four stages of portion control. The amount of carbs, protein and vegetables (fiber) changes each month. The goal is to trigger fat burning mode in the first phase and finally ease the user into a balanced diet to maintain the weight loss. By doing portions you eat in the same portions every time you eat, teaching your stomach to communicate with your brain. After few weeks, your stomach gut system gets used to your portion intake and can make the desired changes to lose weight.

Often, SlimPlate users provide feedback telling us how much they actually under-eat in specific meals (like breakfast) and overeat at dinner. The SlimPlate System corrects this horrible habit and helps them lose weight.

Eating irregularly isn't good for losing weight. It clogs and jams the metabolism.

We always advocate to our patients to control their portions **systematically** and to achieve their goal of losing weight by eating what they like, not by starving or extreme dieting.

That is the right way to use portion control to lose weight effectively for the long-term.

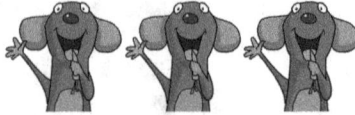

Chapter 11

Fat-Me-Not Success Strategy

Action Plan to Start Now

Here is the promised Fat-Me-Not success plan, your action plan for success. To make it easy to read and follow I have divided the Fat-Me-Not weight loss plan in four parts.

Part I: Action Plan to Start Now

Part II: Overcoming Weight Loss Challenges

Part III: Fine-Tuning Your Weight Loss

Part IV: Smart Exercising to Enhance Weight Loss

This chapter, Part I of the Fat-Me-Not Success Strategy, deals with the very basic rules you need to start following right away to lose weight.

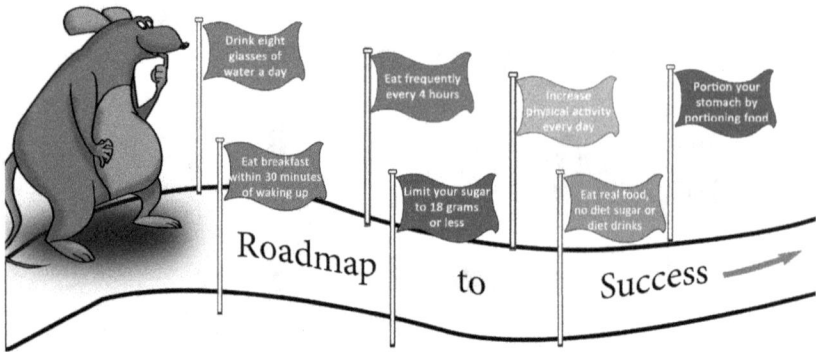

So far we have learned about anatomy and the way our body functions, what obesity can do to the body, and the right way to lose weight.

Now we come to the action plan: what are we going to do to lose weight.

The Fat-Me-Not success plan is simple, but highly effective. Remember, the right weight loss has to be easy, has to allow real food, and develops a lifetime habit.

As the plan is easy, you might think less of its power. All these steps are based on the science that I have previously gone through. If you do it, you'll reap long-term benefits with ease. I have added additional tips for those of you using the SlimPlate System, so you can synchronize Fat-Me-Not weight loss plan in this book with your SlimPlate System.

It is time to start! So let's get going.

There are 7 rules and all need to be followed. Do not pick and choose the ones you will follow because they all work in conjunction. They all need to be in the plan at the same time for the long term.

Rule no. 1: Drink eight glasses of water a day.

Drink eight glasses of water per day. Drink it every time you eat a snack and with meals. With the SlimPlate system, you eat about five times a day, so you'll drink five cups of water. Then you'll drink one cup of water after each meal. This will bring your total to eight cups.

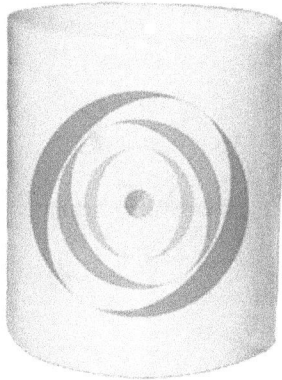

Can you drink more than eight cups of water?
Yes. But drink at least eight cups per day.

Do I need to drink according to the above plan?
You don't need to, but that's the best way to develop the habit. It will also make it easier for you to limit calories. You will feel fuller and more satisfied by drinking a glass of water before meals.

Can I drink other drinks than water?

You can drink other drinks as special drinks; keep a limit of two cups per day in a given cup. For example, you could drink coffee, milk, juice, regular soda, or other soft drinks. Often, drinks are the culprits of weight gain, so I stress that you use 8 oz cups. Those using the SlimPlate System can use the portion cups provided in the set. Use the cold cup for cold drinks and the hot mug for hot drinks.

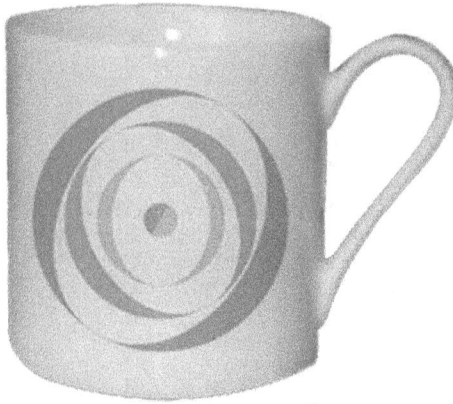

Can diet drinks be consumed?

Not at all. I recommend drinking regular drinks (in appropriate portions) instead of diet drinks. Other than water, you can have black coffee, sparkling water, unsweetened green tea, and fruit-flavored water. But no diet drinks!

What is the benefit of drinking water?

Drinking water and maintaining your body's hydration has many benefits.

1. Lowers energy intake
2. Facilitates long-term weight loss
3. Effectively reduces weight gain
4. Increases metabolic rate by stimulating sympathetic system
5. Water in the body regulates the metabolism
6. Improves the exercise capacity of muscle

Rule no. 2: Eat breakfast within 30 minutes of waking up

Yes! Wake up, brush your teeth and start eating your breakfast before doing anything else. Do not prolong the night long fast so your body does not switch to fat saving mode when you actually eat.

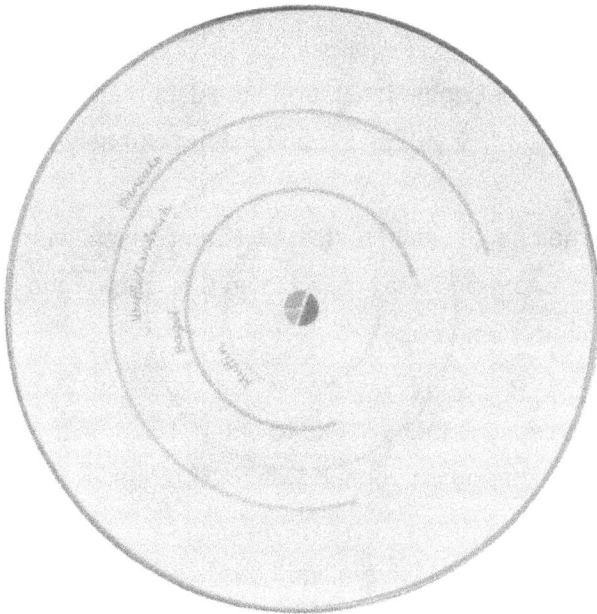

What can you eat for breakfast?

Either of these:

1. You can eat cereal, oatmeal, or grits in a 12 oz bowl
   (If you have SlimPlate System you can use the cereal bowl.)

2. You can eat any of your favorite breakfast carbohydrates, including pancakes, muffins, bagels, and waffles as long as you can carve them into the following diameters. (Again SlimPlate system users can eat on the provided breakfast plate using the appropriate cutters in the set)
   a) Muffin = 2 inch diameter
   b) Bagel = 3 inch diameter
   c) Waffle = 4 inch diameter
   d) Pancake = 5 inch diameter

3. You can eat eggs, toast, and breakfast meats like sausage and bacon; any three in combination can be your breakfast.

4. Some people like breakfast-style smoothies, with yogurt, fruit, and granola, all mixed in an 8 oz cup (or the SlimPlate System's cold cup).

5. Anything else that you like to eat, but portion it or use the SlimPlate portion cups, bowls and cutters.

Why it should be within the first hour of waking up?

We want to improve our metabolism and increase our calorie expenditure. Also we want to prevent our body from switching into fat saving mode.

As we wake up, the body is ready to start; growth hormones, thyroid hormones, cortisol, and other hormones are ready to jump-start our powerhouse. We want to fuel it right to make maximum use of it.

What if we don't have time in the morning?

Take it to go on the way. Items no. 1 and 3 above, can be easy to carry. But make sure you have breakfast every day.

I can't eat breakfast in the morning; I feel too nauseated to eat; I'm not hungry.

If you are not hungry in the morning when you wake up, there is something abnormal about your metabolism. I commonly see this with my obese patients. They are so used to not eating breakfast that they actually feel sick if they try to eat in the early morning.

Start out with warm milk or something soft like boiled eggs or yogurt, and slowly escalate to eating what you want down the line.

Once you start eating breakfast, you will get used to eating breakfast and it will become easier and easier.

Rule no. 3: Eat frequently, approximately every four hours. Or five times a day.

Everyday eat correct portions of breakfast, lunch, dinner and two snacks spread in between.

Why eat so many times?

You don't want your brain to think that there is scarcity of food and access to food is unpredictable for the body. Because then the brain will tell your body to start storing fat instead of consuming it and you won't lose inches from your waist.

This is why, in the SlimPlate weight loss program, you eat five times a day.

Is there flexibility?

Choose a plan according to your daily schedule. In order to eat five times a day, eat breakfast, lunch, dinner, and two snacks. Depending on when you wake up, you can alter the snack time. I'm a night owl, so I chose the night owl plan and add my second snack after dinner. If you're an early bird, place your first snack in between breakfast and lunch.

Eat 5 times a day!
Choose Your Option

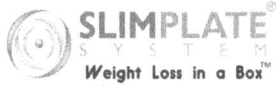

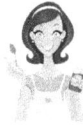

Early Bird

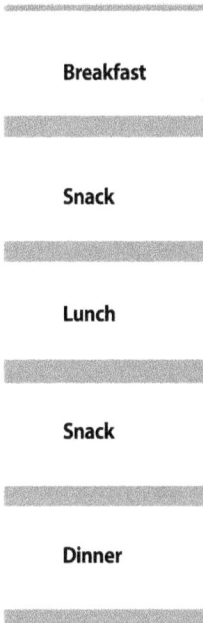

Breakfast

Snack

Lunch

Snack

Dinner

Night Owl

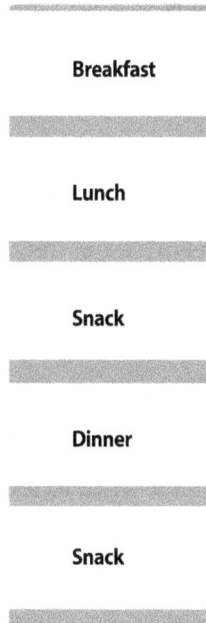

Breakfast

Lunch

Snack

Dinner

Snack

Drink plenty of water a day

Limit other beverages to 2 cups per day

Drink a glass of water before each meal and snack

In our body, it isn't the heart, the brain, or the skin that spends the most calories, but rather the gut system — it spends 30-35% of the total calories spent by the body. So make it work for you five times a day.

Do you want to know more?

The small muscle, which takes food from your mouth all the way to the rectum; the juices from the mouth to the rectum; enzymes that digest big chunks of food to make it into invisible particles; the process of taking nutrients into the body system across the border lining the gut — it creates, replenishes, and makes the participants of the digestive system the biggest energy spender.

If you want to lose weight, you have to ask your gut to work the best for you. Eating frequently and eating real food is a workout for the gut system.

This is why you feel warm after eating; your gut is working out for you. Be smart: eat frequently and lose weight.

Can you eat more than five times?

Surprisingly the answer is yes. I have done this in my practice. Sometimes, my obese patients, above 300 pounds, need to have more calories. So I had to add a third snack to let them eat six times a day. The idea is not to feel hungry so our body does not feel it has to save calories as fat.

If you feel hungry despite eating as instructed, you can add another snack.

Often, stunted weight loss can be thus sped up in obese patients.

What if I can only eat three or four times a day?

Add additional meal or snack to make it five. There are multiple ways to easily eat snacks. Ten large nuts or twenty peanuts or pistachios, fresh fruit in SlimPlate fruit saucer, or a cup of coffee with cream and sugar are my usual mid-afternoon snacks.

Rule no. 4: Limit your sugar to 18 grams or less at a time

When does it apply?

This applies to items for which you cannot measure or use the SlimPlate System tool — mostly packaged snacks. I want you to be able to enjoy anything that you like, including a candy bar or a bag of cookies. Just portion them appropriately. There are various kinds of packaged snacks containing different ingredients.

Check the sugar content (not carbohydrate content). For example if you're eating a candy bar, take a look at the sugar content on the food label. If a candy bar has 36 gram of sugar in a serving size, then you can cut it in half so that you don't exceed 18 grams. You can eat half of the bar now and the other half later.

How do you portion chocolate?

It is not practical for me to detail correct portion sizes of all snacks in this book, as it will make it bulky. I will refer you to mobile app called SlimPlate. Download it free and go to the 'food suggestion' section. There is a chocolate section that suggests how to portion different chocolate brands. This way, you don't lose your weight loss plan but are still able to enjoy your sweet treats.

Here is the link: https://itunes.apple.com/us/app/slimplate-weight-loss-lose/id591827702?mt=8

Here is the QR code for iPhone and Android.

How do you portion cheese?

This is also listed in the SlimPlate mobile app.

In the SlimPlate mobile app, choose your cheese portion to stay on course with your weight loss plan.

Can I really eat chips?

Yes! You can.

When you eat fruit, chips, popcorn, or any other snack items, just eat one handful only. Those with SlimPlate System, place them in the fruit saucer (snack bowl) to correctly portion them. As long as you portion them in the SlimPlate fruit saucer, it should be fine to consume. Nobody should tell you chips are bad. They aren't bad; they just need to be portioned. Large portion of fruits may also slow your weight loss, even though fruit is good for you.

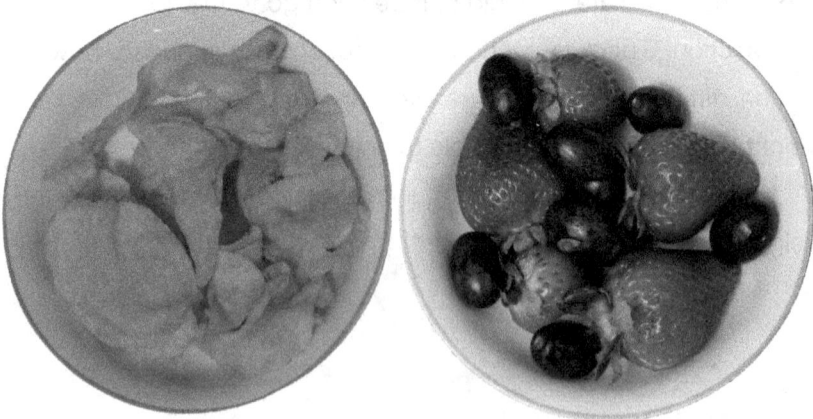

This reminds me of a story of this sweet patient of mine.

I have a very sweet male, Greek patient. When he talks, his arms swing wide as he gestures. Every time, he gestures with enthusiasm — both arms.

He said to me that because of his health, he was watching his diet. He didn't eat meat; he'd given up pork and sausages, and only ate fruits and vegetables.

He said that he knew fruits were good for him, and he'd eaten a watermelon as a snack before coming to see me.

The problem was that his weight bothered him. His weight didn't budge even though he'd eaten nothing but fruit and vegetables for several months.

He asked me to check him and to take his blood, because he was sure that something was wrong.

I knew him and his family well; they were a well-travelled, well-educated family and took care of themselves. He had recently had an unexplained seizure-like episode and had discovered he was diabetic. The entire family was shocked by his illness and they all became more health cautious than ever.

I asked what kinds of fruits and vegetable he ate. I also wasn't sure at that point what was going on. He had pretty much changed his lifestyle without seeing any results, and I knew he must be disappointed.

He did not drink any soft or hard drinks. He had become a vegetarian and, after a few months, there should have been some positive results.

With nothing to go by I asked him how much of a watermelon he had before coming here.

He swung open his arms again until his fingers touched in front of his belly, showing me the size of the watermelon he ate each time.

Having got the answer, I smiled.

I would not have thought that he was eating an entire watermelon at a time, calling it his snack.

One slice of watermelon may be good. May be two slices. But definitely not the whole watermelon. But he really thought he could eat a whole watermelon everyday as a snack.

Basically, it was too much of a good thing turning into a bad thing.

Though he thought he was doing well by restricting his meat and fat intake, he was still consuming a great deal of sugar at one time.

Fruit is good for the body; they are nutrient and vitamin rich, but we have to portion them too. You can have fruit 2-3 times as a snack, but eating fruit like a whole watermelon will harm rather than help you.

Do you know why we need to portion the sugar *intake each time?*

Sugar (glucose) is easily absorbed and instantly rises up in the blood. Then it stimulates sharp rise in insulin secretion. Insulin then turns the sugar in the blood into fat. This is why it is undesirable to eat a large portion of sugar at one time. It should be spread out over time. It is okay to eat one cookie for each snack, but you don't want to eat two large cookies for one snack. It will make your sugar rise and your body will start saving fat rather than burning it.

Rule no. 5: Limit your drink calories; Avoid diet drinks

Portion regular drinks. 8oz at a time not more than once a day.

Artificial sweeteners, including natural sweeteners, are to be avoided, as they are known to cause rebound craving of sweets and calories. I encourage everyone to eat real food and real drinks in portion.

Diet sugar can make your metabolism do the opposite of what you want. I want you to have regular sugar; it may give you extra calories, but it won't make your metabolism chaotic like artificial sweetener can.

Artificial sweetener can damage your metabolism and thus weight loss by creating craving and binging. It also disturbs normal metabolism by clogging and jamming it.

Rule no. 6: Eat real food (rather than egg beaters, protein bars or shakes)

I would encourage you to move toward healthy eating as you lose weight. It will benefit you, not only in trying to lose weight, but also in terms of your overall health. It only takes a few seconds of your time, and when you change these small things in your home, you and your family will get used to this new healthy life style in no time.

- Change your cooking oil to vegetable oil or olive oil, with no cholesterol.
- Change your dairy products to 2% or less fat.
- Change your sugar to brown, large crystal sugar from fine white sugar

Don't eat protein bars, or shakes as meal replacements. These are artificial foods and may be lower in calories than your real food; but do not give your gut a work out so the net result is that you get more calories from them than from the real food.

Don't keep artificial sweeteners in your home. If you run into a diet drink once in a while, it's not the end of the world, but daily consumption of artificial sweeteners can sabotage your weight loss efforts.

Eating real food has many benefits:

1. Increases the thermic effect of food and improves energy expenditure
2. Improves metabolism and spends energy
3. Improves satiety and satisfies the brain
4. Cuts food cravings

Rule no. 7: Portioning automates the weight-loss process for a lifetime

How do you automate portion control?

A slice of bread, steak, and vegetable soup make a satisfying meal without making you feel like you're in a weight loss program. Stir-fried vegetables, chicken, and a portion of rice make a good, hearty meal, yet it's kept in nice portions to keep you in good shape. It is tough to talk about exact portions without a visual plate in front of you. But I will encourage you to look at pictures of SlimPlate System at www.slimplatesystem.com to get an idea.

As you see in the set of SlimPlate system, the plates are exactly the same size; only the ingredients change. The SlimPlate System set takes you through four steps of portion control.

You can build a sandwich with any meat or vegetables, but the cutter will size them into same size every time. That is what we need in order to learn and form long-term habits to keep the weight off.

What is the benefit of portion control?

There are many benefits. You have learned how different diets can cause a relapse in weight gain.

In the portion control weight loss, you eat the same portions for a lifetime. You eat real food on a well-balanced plate (maintenance plate). You are all set from day one to prevent a relapse into weight gain.

These plates help you to form good eating habits for life. You eat real, balanced food, so your gut hormones won't return to the Fat-Me-Yes storm and drag you into relapse.

Can I really eat anything that I want and cook in different style?

You can really eat any kind of food from the entire world and experiment with different ethnic cooking styles. I also encourage you to eat good food as long as it fits the plates. Often you'll be surprised you eat very little due to the fear that you may not lose weight. But it creates the starvation mode in your body and instead of losing weight; it can actually make you gain weight.

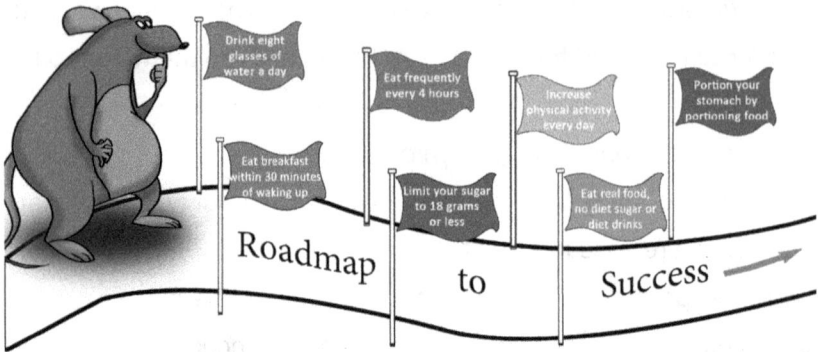

Drink eight glasses of water a day

Eat frequently every 4 hours

Increase physical activity every day

Portion your stomach by portioning food

Eat breakfast within 30 minutes of waking up

Limit your sugar to 18 grams or less

Eat real food, no diet sugar or diet drinks

Roadmap to Success

The SlimPlate System Way

For those who are not familiar with the SlimPlate System, let me give some background on it. We designed the SlimPlate System based on the very principles discussed in this book. The goal has been to create a complete dinnerware with visual cues and make the Fat-Me-Not diet easy to follow. People from all over the US have been using it. It can be ordered at www.slimplatesystem.com.

The first step in the SlimPlate weight loss program is to use the 'Inspire' plate for either lunch or dinner. In this first plate, you don't get to eat starch in one meal of the day. You can have cereals at breakfast; you can have a sandwich for lunch; you can even have chips as a snack. But for one meal of the day, in first step, you can't eat starch. This step lasts a month and is designed to trigger fat burning mode.

Starch includes rice, pasta, potatoes, and bread. Cutting back starch in one meal of the day in the beginning helps you get to fat-burning mode much faster.

If it is a stir-fried mixed dish with chicken and vegetables, you don't have to split the meat and vegetables to place them on the plate. Just let it cover up to the rim for men and the inner circle for women.

The level of the food is an eye estimate of the rim level of the plate. A chicken drumstick is high above the rim of the plate, so leave some space in the meat section. Make your best guess. If you eat a bit extra, it is okay too. No need to sweat.

In the second step, after the end of first month, it is time to use the second portion plate 'Savvy' which allows introduction of carbs back in to the one meals. In the third month 'Savvy' plate is switched to 'Master' portion plate and finally after completion of weight loss program user switches to 'Maintenance' plate to maintain the lost weight.

So this is how a portion control system works. It is designed for life. So there is no end to it. Once you start on this path, visual cues guide you and over time train you surreptitiously. Healthy habits then tiptoe into your life and; before you know most of your bad eating habits are corrected and you become what you always wanted to be: healthy, confident, slim and energetic.

So you have completed the first part of Fat-Me-Not success strategy. There are three more parts to this plan to empower you and make your weight loss effort successful. Keep on reading and applying the knowledge you have gained. This is how I train my patients to lose weight in my weight loss clinic. And I am happy to be able to bring it to you. But don't wait until you are done reading this book, apply what you have learnt right away.

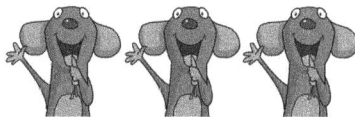

Chapter 12

Fat-Me-Not Success Strategy Part II:

Losing Weight with Challenges

1. *Losing weight with menopause*

2. *Losing weight while on steroids*

3. *Losing weight with mental disabilities*

4. *Losing weight with physical disabilities*

5. *Losing weight with irritable stomach/food allergies*

6. *Losing weight with abnormal thyroid*

7. *Losing weight with sleep disturbance*

8. *Losing weight when nursing/breastfeeding*

9. *Losing weight when in stress*

Losing Weight with Challenges

We all have our own stories and struggles. The previous chapter is for the general public. If you have special conditions that limit your ability to lose weight, I have made an action plan for those special conditions, too.

I have told you many stories about how obesity can affect our bodies and our health.

It is not only a few percent of obese people that are unhealthy. All obese people are, in one way or another, unhealthy at some level. Some may have limited mobility; some may get cancer; some may get heart disease; some may suffer from stroke; some may get sleeping disorders; and some may get many diseases at once.

As weight gain isn't sudden, people get used to the obesity effect on their bodies. It's like you just don't realize what you have lost and even pain and suffering feels like it is supposed to be like this.

For example, I had one patient who hadn't been in the shower for fourteen years. She was big enough that she couldn't stand in the shower, so she started self-bathing with a washcloth. The problem was that she couldn't reach down to her legs, so they remained unwashed. Then one day, she developed an infection in her legs; that was how I found out she hadn't been washing them. Dead skin flakes and the dust on her legs were hardening the skin on her legs because she wasn't able to wash the area. But she did not realize not being able to take a shower is not normal.

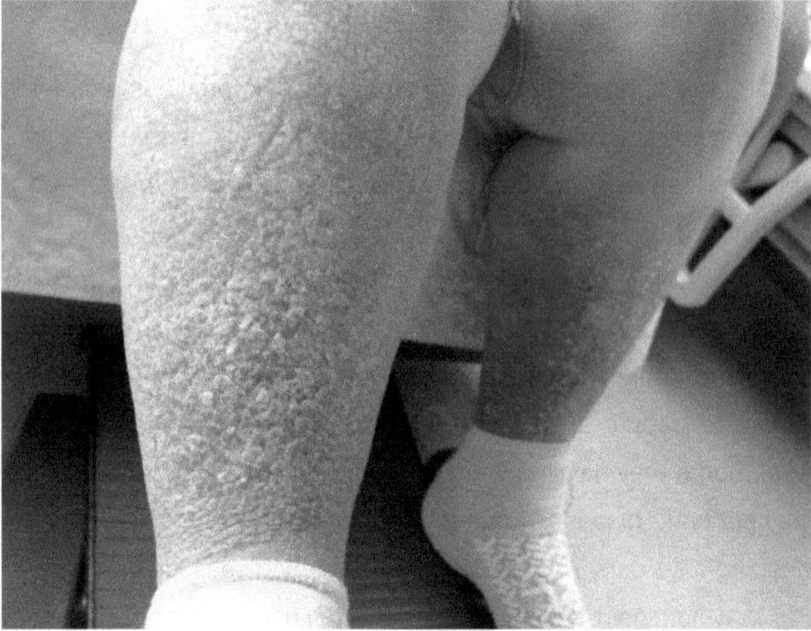

The culprit was obesity. If she hadn't been obese, she wouldn't have had a bad back and would have been able to reach down to her legs.

But she did not realize that she couldn't shower because she was obese; she just put the blame on her bad back.

There is a lot about "fat-shaming" in the media. The media's arguments make the rest of us confused. Should we all be fat-proud?

I am the physician coach for the overweight and the obese. I know how they feel and how they suffer. I am with them as they struggle and succeed; I am their troubleshooter.

Everyone wants to be healthy and pain free. Move freely, sleep better, feel energetic, and not have to take medications. Everyone wants to live longer, to take care of his or her children and enjoy life.

I have a strong point to make here. Fat shaming or being fat-proud neither is good. Being obese is nothing to be ashamed of or to be proud of. It is just a disease like any other such as diabetes, or high blood pressure etc. The point is that you need to lose weight to achieve a healthy weight that will allow you to stay healthy for the rest of your life. We all have one life and we should strive to enjoy it fully.

I repeat this topic again and again, because until we know that we need to lose weight, until we accept that obesity is unhealthy, we can't go further.

Once we set our mind to it, the rest will follow suit. And here are some sticky situations when losing weight is not that easy.

1. *Losing weight with menopause*
2. *Losing weight while on corticosteroids*
3. *Losing weight with mental disabilities*
4. *Losing weight with physical disabilities*
5. *Losing weight with irritable stomach/food allergies*
6. *Losing weight with abnormal thyroid*
7. *Losing weight with sleep disturbance*
8. *Losing weight when nursing/breastfeeding*
9. *Losing weight in stress*

Losing weight with menopause

Menopausal age is actually a golden age for women. Women aren't the only ones to lose hormones; men do as well. It is called Andro-pause in men.

I always tell men and women at this age that they've reached their golden age and that I actually look forward to it.

I look forward to the age of fifty because by this age, we have experienced life, richness, poverty, hard work, sorrow, happiness, luck, fortune, death, birth, losses, and gains.

We would have seen it all and have gotten enough of life to be able to continue on to the next step of life.

We can shape our lives how we want. If you want a peaceful life, go for it. If you want a successful life, strive for it. If you want a family life, work for it. We really can't fall back from where we are already.

When I reach this golden age, I'd like my life to be peaceful, and I'd like to be mentally and physically healthy.

Now we just need to achieve what we want in life.

For those at the post-reproductive point of their lives:

1. Eat a balanced diet; avoid fad diets that put you through stressful cycles of weight loss and rebound weight gain.

2. Stay hydrated by drinking at least eight glasses of water per day.

3. Do thirty minutes of exercise or physical activity per day.

4. Use the portion control way to lose weight and maintain it, as this is a healthy way of losing weight. You can combine the SlimPlate System with the Fat-Me-Not success plan.

5. Discuss hormone replacement therapy with your doctor (for both men and women).

6. Take vitamins, including multivitamins, B12, vitamin D, folic acid, and calcium.

---

7. Get an annual physical from the doctor even if you don't have any diseases.
8. Keep stress to a minimum. (More to come on handling stress)
9. Avoid unnecessary antibiotic use.
10. Discuss your medications with your doctor, as they may cause weight gain; discuss switching to weight-neutral alternatives.
11. Sleep well between 11pm and 4am, or longer.
12. Follow **all** tips, not just some of them, for success.

A balanced diet should include all macronutrients. It should promote protein intake because that help improve lean muscle mass. It should limit sugar intake without eliminating it. Take this advice seriously. Even we designed SlimPlate System based on these principles. Eating five times a day, with appropriate portion control, will not only help you lose weight but will also promote energy, nutrition, and overall wellbeing.

Hormone replacement therapy for men and women should be discussed with your own doctors at length.

The benefits to hormone replacement therapy, which include estrogen and progesterone treatment for women and testosterone replacement for men, are well known, as are their undesired side effects. Only your doctor can tell if it is right for you.

Check your hormone levels to see where you stand. Often, saggy arms and a pouting belly may be the sign that your body is lacking hormones as well as lacking well-balanced nutrition.

At the age of fifty, you should start taking vitamins, multivitamins, vitamin D, and calcium. Any other over-the-counter medications that you take should be discussed with your doctor.

Losing weight while on corticosteroids

Corticosteroids, whether taken intravenously, intra-nasally, or by oral ingestion, can hinder your weight loss and even cause undesirable weight gain.

Often, if you have inflammatory diseases like rheumatoid arthritis, uncontrolled asthma, inflammatory bowel disease, or chronic obstructive pulmonary disease, you may need intermittent or chronic sustained steroids.

It can be frustrating when you're working hard to lose weight but have to be on steroids.

If you're on steroids:

1. Stay on a regular exercise plan, even if it's only walking 30 minutes a day.
2. Limit your salt intake; don't add salt and avoid salty food.
3. Drink plenty of water at least 8 cups per day.
4. Limit your sugar intake. Delete sugary drinks from your Fat-Me-Not plan. Trade out your snacks for 10 large nuts, yogurt, and boiled eggs. If you usually drink two cups of special drinks with SlimPlate portion cups, you should replace these with water.
5. Eat well-balanced meals, more proteins and veggies but less carbs.

6. Add fifteen minutes of yoga or a similar flexibility exercise to your exercise routine.
7. Frequently rinse and gargle with saltwater to avoid fungal infections.
8. Avoid unnecessary use of antibiotics during steroid use.
9. Talk to your doctor to change steroids from oral ingestion to a local administration such as a nasal spray, if possible.
10. Minimize the dosage as much as possible and lower the dosage as your symptoms improve. Never abruptly stop taking the steroids, however.
11. Keep stress to a minimum.
12. Discuss your medications with your doctor, as they may cause you to gain weight; consider changing to weight-neutral alternatives.
13. Take multivitamins, including B12, vitamin D, calcium, folic acid, and chromium*.
14. Sleep well between 11pm to 4am, or longer.
15. Follow **all** tips, not just some of them, in order to have the best success.

*Chromium is in common foods, including potatoes, wholegrain breads, and cereals. You can replace chromium safely by choosing chromium-rich foods, as the side effects of chromium overuse are common and may not be noticed, as we don't usually check these blood levels.

It is tough to be on steroids while trying to lose weight, but the above tips will get you through it.

Losing weight with mental disabilities

These are the challenges we face in our daily lives. Most medications used for various mental disorders actually make people gain weight. When they aren't in a balanced frame of mind, they aren't able to take care of themselves in a way that they're able to lose weight; which makes the situation worse.

We have to cut the chain of this cycle from one end.

The medications that can make you gain weight can be seen below. Discuss these with your doctor and mention clearly that you are trying to lose weight. Request to be switched to an alternative anything that causes you to gain weight or, if that isn't possible, if you can be put on a lower dose.

Psychotropic
1. Olanzapine
2. Lithium
3. Clozaril (clozapine)
4. Zyprexa (olanzapine)
5. Remeron (mirtazapine)
6. Seroquel (quetiapine)
7. Depakote (divalproex)
8. Paxil (paroxetine)
9. Tricyclics (nortriptyline, imipramine, doxepin)

Available alternative weight-neutral medications include:

1. Weight-neutral antidepressants
    a) Lexapro (escitalopram)
    b) Zoloft (sertraline)
    c) Prozac (fluoxetine)
    d) Wellbutrin (bupropion)

2. Weight-neutral antipsychotics
    a) Aripiprazole (abilify)
    b) Asenapine (saphrys)
    c) Lurasidone (latuda)
    d) Ziprasidone (Geodon)

There are many medicine alternatives to choose from for most mental disorders, including depression, bipolar, seizure disorders, and schizophrenia. You should discuss these further with your doctor or psychiatrist, and you should not abruptly stop any medication.

You don't need to start your weight loss journey when you're actively being treated for a psychiatric condition, but you can be cautious about side effects of medications, including weight gain. This way, weight gain won't burden you further when the active problem is under control.

Once a mental problem is under control, you can start a healthy and long-term weight loss plan using portion-control weight loss program.

- Avoid yo-yo dieting.
- Avoid extreme dieting.
- Avoid starvation.
- Avoid anything that you can't do for a lifetime.

The above techniques I ask you to avoid is because they will unsettle your achievement of a balanced mood. It can significantly harm people who need help with mental health.

Either you can monitor your portions or you can use the SlimPlate weight loss program to keep your calorie intake in check; it will serve as a constant reminder to eat balanced and healthily, and you will be able to form good habits for the long-term.

Mentally disabled patients in particular should be in a stable environment, with stable food, and a routine of eating; this will get them into healthy habits rather than into rebounding habits.

Always check with doctors about the stability of hormones in the body. Check lab tests, including thyroid hormones, steroid hormones, sex hormones, electrolytes, and vitamins.

Together with your mental health doctor, primary care doctor, and therapist, you can promote your weight loss results and a stable mental state.

If you suffer from mental disabilities:
1. Eat five times a day.
2. Drink eight glasses of water a day.
3. Eat in the right portions or use the SlimPlate System portion cups, cutters, and plates.
4. Limit sugar intake during snacks to less than 18 grams. This only applies to snacks for which you can't use the SlimPlate snack bowl .i.e. if you are using the system. For example you should only eat half of a candy bar with a sugar content of 36 grams.
5. Avoid artificial and natural sweeteners. Use cane sugar.

6. Use 8 oz cups for soft drinks or use SlimPlate cups and mugs.

7. For eating out, use the SlimPlate app for drinks, alcohol, and menu choices. It is free to download.

8. Do any activity that can make you warm and sweat for thirty minutes.

9. Avoid unnecessary antibiotics use.

10. Discuss your medications with your doctor, as they may cause weight gain; if possible switch to weight-neutral alternatives.

11. Take multivitamins, B12, vitamin D, calcium, and folic acid.

12. Minimize stress.

13. Sleep well between 11pm to 4am, or longer.

14. Follow **all** tips, not just some of them, in order to maximize success.

Losing weight with physical disabilities

There's a popular belief that people with physical disabilities can't lose weight.

Not only can they lose weight, but also they need to do so in order to improve their disabilities.

Any time I discuss weight loss with my physically disabled patients, they wrongly attribute their physical disabilities as the reason they haven't been able to be active, as the reason that they've become so big.

You have to understand one thing about me here. If I had a supernatural power, or if I were granted one wish, I would wish for everyone in the world to be their healthy weight and free from suffering.

I understand my patients perfectly; they don't feel good about how they look or how much they weigh. They know their weight is the reason for their high blood pressure, their diabetes. They feel helpless to the point they don't think there's anything they can do about it.

In the media, we always see upbeat, nice, lean people doing fitness and getting active, marching along on a treadmill, sweating and smiling the whole time. My physically disabled patients don't feel they can possibly be like them, not when they can barely walk from their bed to a chair.

So they become used to the fact that weight loss is not for them; it's for people who can walk on a treadmill.

But it is not true. The top ten most important things to losing weight are:

1. Diet
2. Diet
3. Diet
4. Diet
5. Diet
6. Diet
7. Diet
8. Diet
9. Diet
10. Exercise

Diet changes the weight control system in our body by altering hormones and the microbiome as we discussed in previous chapter. This in turn changes calorie intake, eating behavior, calorie expenditure, and ultimate metabolism. All of this together makes us lose weight.

This is my favorite thing to tell my patients. They light up.

I tell them to forget about the exercise that they can't do, and to focus on the diet that they **can** do, nine times out of ten. Exercise is only one out of ten times.

I get them to focus on the nine-time thing and to forget about the one-time thing.

We have helped many of patients lose their wheelchairs, canes, pain, and illnesses, despite the fact that they are physically disabled.

For those with physical disabilities:
1. Eat five times a day.
2. Drink eight glasses of water a day.
3. Eat in the right portions or use SlimPlate portion cups, cutters, and plates to make it easy for you to manage portions.
4. Limit sugar intake during snacks to less than 18 grams. This only applies to snacks for which you can't use the SlimPlate snack bowl. For example, you should only eat half of a candy bar with a sugar content of 36 grams.
5. Avoid artificial and natural sweeteners. Use cane sugar
6. Use the SlimPlate cups and mugs for drinks other than water.

7. For eating out, use the SlimPlate app for drinks, alcohol, and menu choices. It is free to download.

8. Do any activity that can make you warm and sweat for thirty minutes. For example, move your arms, tap on the floor, push up out of your wheelchair, do hand-squeezing exercises, or engage in water activity.

9. Rather than depend solely on oral pain medications, use other pain control methods such as topical applications, heating pads, injections, stretching, or physical therapy.

10. Avoid unnecessary antibiotics use.

11. Discuss your medications with your doctor, as they may cause weight gain; if possible switch to weight-neutral alternatives.

12. Take multivitamins, B12, vitamin D, calcium, glucosamine, and folic acid.

13. Minimize stress.

14. Sleep well between 11pm and 4am, or longer.

15. Follow **all** tips, not just some of them, in order to maximize success.

Losing weight with irritable stomach/food allergies

I have a few patients with various gastrointestinal problems, like food allergies, weak stomachs, irritable bowel problems, and food intolerances.

Weight loss is possible with all type of problems and limitations. The key is to focus on what you can do, rather than what you can't do

- There are people who can't eat chicken.

- There are people who can't tolerate dairy products.
- There are people who can't tolerate vegetables.
- There are people who can't tolerate dry beans.
- There are people who can't tolerate many of the above.

So we don't focus on the food that we can't tolerate. We choose what we like and what we can eat.

Make a list of what you can eat. Divide them into protein, carbs and veggies. Then choose their portions or put it on the SlimPlate portion plates, if you have one. For example, if you can't eat chicken, place beef or seafood in the protein area. If you can't eat broccoli, place green beans in the green section. If you can't eat gluten, eat rice or gluten-free grains in the blue section.

Often, patients cure their problems with regular eating habits.

I had a patient who was frequently constipated for months, keeping her from eating regularly. No kidding. I put her on a balanced diet with the SlimPlate System. Her constipation was cured.

It isn't magic. Research has found that changing the gastrointestinal flora with the food that we eat actually alters the gastrointestinal immune system. This is why, when you eat regularly and eat real, organic food (without chemicals, growth hormones, or growth-promoting antibiotics used in meat), you can improve your gastrointestinal defense system and cure the illnesses you've been suffering from.

I have patients who resolved their diet-induced diarrhea by eating a balanced meal with real food, with the SlimPlate System.

If you have food allergies or intolerances:

1. Choose organic food.
2. Choose 100% wholegrain bread unless you have gluten sensitivity.
3. Choose vegetables grown without chemicals.
4. Test for gluten sensitivity. If the test is positive, switch to rice and gluten-free substitutes.
5. Test for lactose intolerance.
6. Test for immunoglobulin deficiency.
7. Avoid use of antibiotics.
8. Eat five times a day.
9. Drink eight glasses of water a day.
10. Eat in the right portions or use the SlimPlate System portion cups, cutters, and plates.
11. Limit sugar intake during snacks to less than 18 grams. This only applies to snacks for which you can't use the SlimPlate snack bowl. For example, you should only eat half of a candy bar with a sugar content of 36 grams.
12. Avoid artificial and natural sweeteners.
13. Use 8 oz cups to drink soft drinks or use the SlimPlate cups and mugs.
14. Take multivitamins, B12, vitamin D, calcium, and folic acid.
15. Minimize stress.
16. Sleep well between 11pm and 4am, or longer.
17. Follow all tips, not just some of them, in order to maximize success.

Losing weight with abnormal thyroid

Thyroid disorder is quite common in women and it can affect your weight loss efforts.

1. Check your hormone levels regularly. If they are at a stable level, check it at least twice a year. If you're still adjusting your hormone levels, you may need to check it more frequently.

2. Be proactive. If you have a female relative with low thyroid levels, you may need to have it checked too

3. Use iodine-fortified salt. Some sea salt has limited iodine.

4. Eat five times a day.

5. Drink eight glasses of water a day.

6. Eat in the right portions or use the SlimPlate portion cups, cutters, and plates.

7. Limit sugar intake during snacks to less than 18 grams. This only applies to snacks for which you can't use the SlimPlate snack bowl. For example you should only eat half of a candy bar with a sugar content of 36 grams.

8. Avoid artificial and natural sweeteners. Use cane sugar.

9. Use 8 oz cups to drink soft drinks or use the SlimPlate cups and mugs.

10. For eating out, use the SlimPlate app for drinks, alcohol, and menu choices. It is free to download.

11. Do any activity that can make you warm and sweat for thirty minutes.

12. Rather than depend solely on oral pain medications, use other pain control methods such as topical applications, heating pads, injections, stretching, or physical therapy.
13. Avoid unnecessary antibiotics use.
14. Discuss your medications with your doctor, as they may cause weight gain; if possible switch to weight-neutral alternatives.
15. Take multivitamins, B12, vitamin D, calcium, glucosamine, and folic acid.
16. Minimize stress.
17. Sleep well between 11pm and 4am, or longer.
18. Follow **all** tips, not just some of them, in order to maximize success.

Losing weight with sleep disturbance

Third-shift workers face additional challenges to shed extra weight.

I advise my patients who work at night and sleep during the day to be on regular eating schedule.

For example, if they sleep during the day on weekdays, they would start/pace with breakfast, lunch, snack, dinner, and snacks from the time they wake up, which would usually be around 2 or 3pm.

Over weekends, they return to sleeping at night and being awake during the day, while resuming an eating schedule beginning when they wake up, around 7-8am, with breakfast, lunch, snacks, and dinner.

Night shift workers are prone to chronic sleep deprivation and circadian misalignment; this can, in turn, cause obesity and resistance to weight loss.

Day and night shift workers have some circadian misalignment between weekdays (working days) and weekends (off days).

If you're a night shift worker:

1. Take over-the-counter melatonin in 1, 2, or 3mg before going to sleep. Melatonin helps with good-quality sleep and helps you feel rested. Start with lower doses and then increase, as higher doses of melatonin may make you feel sleepy.

2. Keep the light bright at night when you're working to stimulate the alert center in your brain.

3. When you sleep in the day, keep the room completely dark.

4. Caffeinated, unsweetened drinks, such as black coffee, are helpful at the beginning of the night shift.

5. Avoid sleep deprivation by ensuring a quality 6-8 hours of sleep during the day. Don't get up to do chores before you finish sleeping.

6. Eat five times a day.

7. Drink eight glasses of water a day.

8. Eat in the right portions given in the SlimPlate portion cups, cutters, and plates.

9. Limit sugar intake during snacks to less than 18 grams. This only applies to snacks for which you can't use the SlimPlate snack bowl. You should only eat half of a candy bar with a sugar content of 36 grams.

10. Avoid artificial and natural sweeteners.

11. Use 8 oz cups to drink soft drinks or use the SlimPlate cups and mugs.

12. For eating out, use the SlimPlate app for drinks, alcohol, and menu choices.

13. Do any activity that can make you warm and sweat for thirty minutes.

14. Avoid unnecessary antibiotics use.

15. Discuss your medications with your doctor, as they may cause weight gain; if possible switch to weight-neutral alternatives.

16. Take multivitamins, B12, vitamin D, calcium, and folic acid.

17. Minimize stress.

18. Follow **all** tips, not just some of them, in order to maximize success.

Losing weight when nursing/breastfeeding

As a nursing mother, you can still try to lose weight without affecting the quality of your breast milk or the quantity available to your infant. A nursing mother should drink approximately 8 to 10 eight-ounce glasses of water a day. A mother can produce up to 750 ml (three glasses) of milk for her infant. It should be enough to avoid thirst by drinking regularly; grab a glass of water when nursing.

Your daily calorie intake shouldn't be less than 1500 Cals, even when you're trying to lose weight, in order to maintain breast milk quality and quantity. You should eat about 300 to 500 calories extra than in your pre-baby time.

Limit your fish intake especially fish high in mercury. Swordfish, tilefish, king mackerel, shark, and white tuna all have a high mercury content, but catfish and salmon are both fine, in moderation. The safest is not more than two servings of fish in a week. You can have shrimp.

During nursing, some mothers need multivitamins, iron, B12, folic acid, and calcium with vitamin D. Talk to your doctor and find out if you need supplements.

Remember, millions of women ahead of you have delivered without these additions. Moderation is the key.

In brief:

1. You can try to lose weight while nursing with your diet and safe exercise.
2. You don't need a lot of extra calories and drinks when you're nursing.
3. Well-balanced meals at regular interval will help with weight loss and will help to maintain breast milk quality.
4. If in doubt, add multiple vitamins once daily.
5. Avoid tobacco, alcohol, and recreational drugs.
6. Up to two cups of caffeinated beverages are okay.
7. Ensure sleep efficiency by sleeping between 11pm and 4am.
8. Eat five times a day.
9. Drink eight glasses of water a day.
10. Eat in the right portions or use the SlimPlate portion cups, cutters, and plates.

11. Limit sugar intake during snacks to less than 18 grams. This only applies to snacks for which you can't use the SlimPlate snack bowl. For example, you should only eat half of a candy bar with a sugar content of 36 grams.

12. Avoid artificial and natural sweeteners.

13. Use 8 oz cups to drink soft drinks or use the SlimPlate cups and mugs.

14. For eating out, use the SlimPlate app for drinks, alcohol, and menu choices.

15. Do any activity you can tolerate that makes you sweat for thirty minutes.

16. Avoid unnecessary antibiotics use.

17. Discuss your medications with your doctor, as they may cause weight gain; if possible switch to weight-neutral alternatives.

18. Take multivitamins, B12, vitamin D, calcium, and folic acid.

19. Minimize stress.

20. Follow **all** tips, not just some of them, in order to maximize success.

Losing weight with stress

Keep your stress to the minimum level.

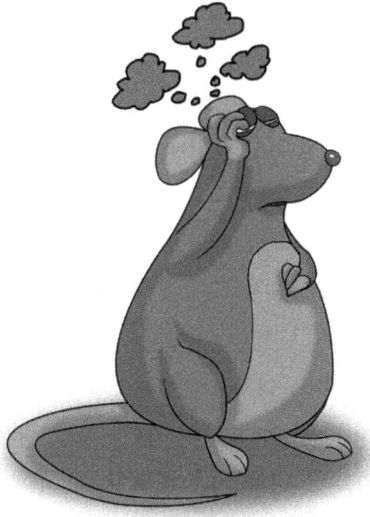

Half of the patients that I see daily in the medical clinic have problems somehow related to stress.

So often as I sit and listen to my patients, I realize that the actual problem isn't medical, but is stress-related.

I often need to treat their blood pressure with mild anxiety medications rather than traditional blood pressure medications.

Often, skin conditions, dizziness, difficulty breathing, chest pain, and obesity are all related to stress.

Stress is a big problem in our lives.

LINDA

Linda was a 56-year-old woman, but she looked like she was seventy-eight. She always looked distressed and anxious, which made her look older.

She was a breast cancer survivor and had a scar on her left chest. Following breast cancer and surgery at forty, her anxiety had gotten worse. Everything haunted her and drove her into a total nervous condition. She ran to the emergency room every fourth night to get checked out. As she couldn't breathe, she had terrible pain on the left side of her chest; with the way she looked, every emergency room doctor thought she was having a heart attack or had a serious blood clot in the lungs.

In the space of ten years, she had more than twenty cardiac catheterizations and over thirty CAT scans of her chest as a result of emergency room visits. Uncountable EKGs and blood tests were done to look for the etiology of her chest pain and difficult breathing. She looked like she could barely get her breath, like she was about to lose her breath. She was placed on a ventilator several times for impending respiratory failure.

I was able to observer her in the clinic, emergency room, and also during her hospital stays during several of her episodes. As a result, I came to realize that her conditions were related to anxiety rather than actual lung or heart disease.

I explained to her that all of these were because of her anxiety. Her many tests didn't show heart disease or blood clots in the lungs over time, so the problem couldn't be any of those conditions. I had to convince her of this fact and advise her to take sedative anxiety medication whenever she developed shortness of breath and chest pain.

Linda was slowly convinced that all of her problems were due to her nerves. I had to get her family and her children all together and make all of them understand the conditions, because when these episodes hit her she looked helpless, terrible, like she was going to die. Her children learned to adapt to this condition and help ease her anxiety attacks.

That is how stress can run your life.

Unfortunately, this case doesn't have a happy ending. We lost her in one of these episodes as a result of complications with a ventilator-dependent respiratory infection; Linda died prematurely.

I have many stories from my time practicing medicine about stress and its effect on the body, but that's for another book.

There are times when we can't get out of our thoughts. One older woman I treated was just too scared to be left alone; she was terrified that death would come while she was alone. Nothing stopped her from these intruding thoughts; much of the latter part of her life, she lived with that fear, until finally death actually got her.

There are things that stress us daily life, as we anticipate that bad things will happen to us.

There are worries about everything, from kids and family to health and money.

It is very easy to say that you shouldn't be stressed, but in practice it's much more difficult to accomplish.

The stress comes in as a storm and destroys the good things you've built up in your life. Sometimes the damage can be unimaginable.

Stress leads to overeating. Overeating can make you stress out again — it's a no-win situation. We already discussed how a wrong diet can make you more stressed.

Stress can lead to long-term anxiety and depression.

Let's look briefly at stress and its consequences, and what we can do to reduce stressful moments without ending up gaining weight.

Some excitement is good, like getting excited to go to work early for a new project. Anticipating problems and planning encounters are good kinds of excitement. But then you start getting anxious about what will happen if the project fails and you start building up thoughts about all of the negative possibilities. This isn't a good thing. It can negatively affect your ability to function, as fear and concerns freeze you. If it happens chronically, then it may even lead one to have an anxiety disorder or even depression.

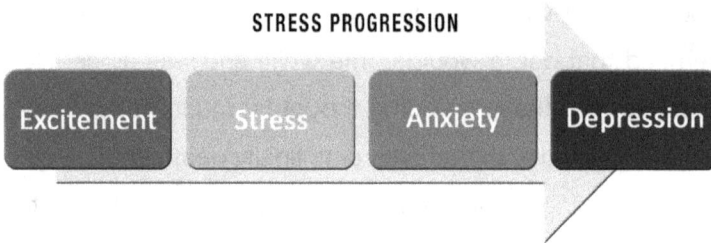

STRESS PROGRESSION

Excitement → Stress → Anxiety → Depression

I sometimes have my patients write down what stresses them daily and categorize them into three groups.

1. Avoid unnecessary stress:

   If traffic causes stress, leave for work early so you can avoid unnecessary stress, or choose another local route if you don't like driving on the freeway. Don't keep fighting stress every day; try to get out of stress mode.

2. Adapt: this may be the perfect answer sometimes. Get used to it. If stress can't be avoided, try adapting and adjusting. Like in relationships, we expect people to change, especially those closest to us. When changes don't happen, we stress over it constantly. Sometimes it

may not be them; we may be the ones that need to adapt and let go of things. Let it go, get used to who the people in your life are, and accept things. We weren't created identically, and that means we're all different. When you let go of little stressful daily things, your life will be much better and more open.

3. Solve it: especially if what's stressing you is something like a task that needs completing. Just face it, deal with it, and get it done. Stop your stress rather than propagate it.

Of course, dealing with stress will take another book altogether. Here, I just want to point out how to stop the stress hormone cascade coming down on us and causing us to overeat.

When we're stressed, our brain stimulates production of a cascade of hormones that make us eat high-fat, high-sugar foods, and we then gain weight. It's good that the brain gets us ready for stressful situations by providing energy, but it also means that your stress system gets stimulated. As long as you stay stressed, you'll end up chronically overeating, resulting in weight gain.

The main point here is that you need to cut off your stress and avoid staying in stress mode.

We can also physically do something to help cut the stress hormone cascade in the body.

It is simple and easy to do and say, but it's harder to practice not staying stressed. However, cutting the stress hormone cascade off from the body is very easy to do.

Every time you find yourself stressed, take a nice deep breath and expand your chest. Repeat this 10-15 times. You'll feel your racing heart and tremulousness fade away as the stress hormones action fades.

Stress cascade in the body is brought on by the sympathetic system and is reversed by the parasympathetic system. Once the sympathetic switch is on, you'll breathe faster, your eyes will widen, your sugar levels will go up, your heart will begin to race, and your blood pressure will rise. It's like you are in fight-or-flight mode.

Parasympathetic is the opposite. Your pupils shrink, your heart beats more slowly, you breathe more slowly, sugar is used for body building rather than used in the blood, your stomach system is absorbing nutrients, there is increased blood flow to your genitalia, and sympathetic action is also dampened. This system is for rest and sleep time.

Both systems are essential for the human body, as we have to be ready to be chased by the tiger as well as be ready for rest and sleep, too.

Imagine being chased by a tiger. This is exactly what it's like for your body if you're always in stress mode. Whenever we find ourselves under stress, we can cut the stress cascade by turning the parasympathetic system back on.

How you can turn on the parasympathetic switch?

Take deep breath expanding your chest, hold your breath, and release slowly.

Or Stay on your knees and elbows for a few minutes. But if it makes you feel weird, just stick with a deep, full breath and hold and release.

There is a side neck massage used to stimulate the para-sympathetic system, but this is primarily done by skilled medical professionals.

This brief deep breathing exercise can be done anywhere, even at work. Sit down and use this as a moment for yourself, to cut the stress cascade out of your body.

Even though this breathing exercise won't take away your stressful situation, it will turn off your body's stress mode.

The bottom line is that you don't want your body to stay in stress mode as this may make you overeat and gain weight.

Another way to cut the stress cascade is to regularly exercise. Doing regular physical activity or exercise reduces your stress hormone response.

I want to share my daily stress-handling technique.

As you can guess, I am also generally fairly stressed. On a daily basis, I deal with my patients' sicknesses and sufferings, life and death. On top of this, I have to be sound and just in order to be able to do my job and help others. I can't be emotional. Can't be extreme. Can't overdo or underdo things. I have to give sound and just advice to others.

In the heat of a busy day, I drink a lot of water, do deep breathing exercise for a minute, and regularly do physical activity. These are my safe guards to keep moving on. Simple? Right!

These simple steps are the most powerful tools to keep you from staying stressed. Practice them daily; you'll find them useful and effective, too.

This is also scientifically proven. Happy breathing, and cut the stress cascade off. This is how people who practice yoga or meditation, or even concentrated golf players improve their stress handling.

If you find yourself stressed, take relaxation breaks throughout the day and practice your breathing exercises.

Take a deep, full breath, hold it for a second, and then release it slowly. Do this ten times. Close your eyes and disconnect from your environment as you do this. This maneuver takes less than five minutes, but it will train you to handle your stress better.

TIPS

- Deep breathing exercise
- Exercise daily
- Volunteer to help the poor, disabled, or elderly
- Read self-help books
- Follow motivational or positive thinking social media posts

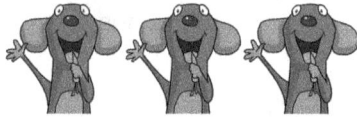

Chapter 13

Understanding Current Weight Loss Treatments

Both Sides of The Coin

Weight Loss Forever: Successful weight loss programs

Remember the three criteria of a good weight loss program

1. Easy to do
2. Allow real food
3. Forms healthy habit for a lifetime

The strategy

1. Limit calorie intake
2. Reset metabolism
3. Maintain it

HCG injection and weight loss: Is it fact or fiction?

We talked about HCG related research before. There is a lot of buzz about HCG (Human Chorionic Gonadotropin) use in medical weight loss programs.

I am frequently asked if I give HCG shots in my weight loss program.

HCG injection use in weight loss was suggested a long time ago. There are multiple weight loss centers outside the US that use HCG injections.

I decided to look into this hype. I researched the literature internationally and domestically and found the following facts regarding HCG:

1. In almost all studies, using HCG injections for weight loss showed no benefits.
2. Most studies didn't show long-term (longer than a few months) effects of weight loss, either.
3. Most studies failed to prove that HCG injections achieve desirable fat mobilization.

So what's all the buzz about HCG?

The original HCG research for weight loss was done with a very low calorie diet (VLCD). Those individuals consumed a maximum of 500 calories per day and were given HCG injections for approximately 1.5 months. They did lose significant weight, but no more than individuals on the VLCD 500 calorie diet alone.

To simplify it: It is very likely that they lost weight because of the low calorie diet rather than because of HCG.

Why there is conflict regarding HCG use in weight loss?

The earth was considered flat once, until we looked at it from different angles. We now have Internet, an open media through which anyone can say anything. Someone might read an old note saying that the earth is flat and then present it as fact.

So are HCG injections any good for weight loss?

Research found that HCG gives you a sense of feeling good. While receiving HCG and VLCD (500 Calories), subjects on HCG could tolerate the misery of a 500 Calorie VLCD better. Essentially, it's a feel-good hormone!

What about body contouring fat loss with HCG?

It isn't true. Multiple studies have looked at this and it doesn't mobilize fat in the desired way.

Does HCG help prevent wrinkles in the skin after losing weight?

It doesn't tighten the skin.

Will you use HCG in your weight loss clinic?

I don't use HCG for losing weight for the following reasons:

1. In my opinion, HCG doesn't help you lose weight. Its possible benefit is to make you feel good when you're on Very Low Calorie Diet (VLCD).

2. I don't support the VLCD of 500 calories a day. Studies show that VLCD cause a greater lean mass loss than fat mass loss.

3. If weight loss is temporary and lasts less than three months, I don't see the point of putting my patients through extreme restrictions and daily shots.

4. Using HCG for its feel-good benefits is pointless, as nobody should feel bad when trying to lose weight. Feeling bad comes from extreme restrictions and doesn't work for the long-term. If you're making it hard to lose weight, you're doing it wrong.

The Orlistat weight loss pill

There are many products on the market that claim to be able to make you lose weight. My patients ask me about these products every day.

One of these products is Orlistat. The TV commercial caught my attention, as it flashed phrases like "FDA approval," "over-the-counter drug," and "fifty percent more reduction". Congratulations to the ad creator.

Let me explain the meaning of these words.

WHAT IS ORLISTAT?

Orlistat is a prescription drug for weight reduction. Prescription-strength Orlistat is 120mg, three times a day. One OTC weight loss product uses 60mg of Orlistat three times a day.

How does it work?

There are several studies looking at Orlistat as an inhibitor of fat digestion for weight reduction. Only one percent of the medication is absorbed into the blood stream; the rest works in the intestines. It blocks the digestive enzymes responsible for breaking down fat and making it suitable for digestion. The dietary fat is not absorbed into the system, resulting in reduced calorie consumption and reduced body weight.

Is it effective?

Let's quantify Orlistat's weight loss effect.

The studies looked at the effect of Orlistat in the weight reduction and maintenance phases. In the weight reduction phase, everyone who was on placebo or on Orlistat was put on lower calorie diets. The studies were done over two years. The first year was for weight reduction and the second year was for weight maintenance.

During the second study, Orlistat 60mg three times a day was used for the maintenance phase where calorie restriction was omitted. Regained weight during maintenance in the Orlistat 120mg and 60mg groups was 3.2 and 4.2 kg, respectively.

> *The bottom line is that Orlistat 120 mg (three times a day) has been shown to promote weight loss of up to 4 kg (8.8 pounds) more than losing weight with diet alone.*

How much weight loss is needed to get FDA approval for a weight-loss drug?

There is no set number. But there is a term called "medically significant weight loss," and a product must reach this in order to get FDA approval.

How much is "medically significant weight loss"?

Weight loss of about five percent of initial body weight can improve your general health and cardiac risk. This is why even a five percent loss from the initial weight is considered medically significant.

A ten to fifteen percent loss is considered a success; more than fifteen percent weight loss is considered very good.

So how do you understand the Orlistat TV ad? Fifty percent weight loss sounds pretty good!

It does sound really good. The TV ad caught my attention the first time I saw it, even though I was feeling sleepy at that time.

Do you understand the advertisement right?

Total weight loss from Orlistat and diet is about 10 kg. Weight loss from diet alone is up to 7 kg. Fifty percent of 7 kg is 3.5 kg.

Basically, the advertisement claims fifty percent more weight loss with Orlistat and diet than diet alone.

It isn't fifty percent of your body weight. It's fifty percent more weight loss with Orlistat than with diet alone, which can be up to 4 kg (8.8 pounds).

What are the side effects of Orlistat? What are its treatment effects?

This is the main difference between doctors and product makers.

As a physician, my first thought is to wonder what the side effects are of the drugs/products.

I guess that comes from the Hippocratic oath that tells us to first do no harm.

As a doctor, I wouldn't polish that as treatment effects, but rather side effects/undesired effects. I want consumers to understand that these side effects are supposed to be weighed against potential benefits.

The listed side effects of Orlistat are as follows:
1. Intestinal borborygmi (stomach rumbling)
2. Abdominal cramps
3. Flatus
4. Fecal incontinence, oily spotting, and flatus with discharge
5. Potential vitamin A, D, E, and K deficiencies as they need fat in order to be absorbed

The occurrence of side effects is up to 30%.

Does Orlistat have any other benefit as a fat blocker?

Orlistat can reduce cholesterol up to ten percent. But remember, there are much more efficacious cholesterol-lowering agents out there; Orlistat isn't suggested for solely cholesterol use.

Phentermine

Patients have asked me if I would take phentermine if I were in their shoes.

Today, I had this friendly question from a patient, asking me if I'd take phentermine if I were obese.

Diet pills carry a "bad" name, particularly phentermine, which is a stimulant-like amphetamine that works in the central nervous system to suppress your appetite and increase metabolism.

Does it help reduce the weight?

It does help with weight loss. But it tends to lose its effectiveness for weight loss when used over a longer period of time. As per my experience and as evidenced in the literature, phentermine helps reduce weight maximally in the first six months. After that, the weight loss effect is less pronounced.

How much weight loss can phentermine achieve?

It actually varies. I do see a larger reduction in larger patients in the initial six months. With diet and exercise, it results in even more weight loss.

For example, Mary tried an exercise program for a month and she lost a pound at the end of it. Then she tried the diet program for a month and lost about two pounds. In the third month, she went to a doctor, got herself a phentermine prescription, and lost only one pound. So she lost about 4 pounds overall.

If she had been on a diet, exercise, and diet pill at the same time, she would have lost far more than the four pounds by the end of the first month, sometimes even up to 20-40 pounds. Diet, exercise, and diet pills together work in **synergy**. A simple pill by itself is not the answer to weight loss.

Does phentermine cause tolerance, dependence, or addiction?

Be warned: phentermine is a scheduled substance and can cause all of the above. Its efficacy can go down as it is used for a longer time, as patients build up tolerance. As it does cause euphoria, people sometimes can get hooked on the higher energy level feeling, leading to addiction. But I haven't seen patients getting addicted to these medications, unlike benzodiazepine (alprazolam, ativan, etc.). Part of the reason may be that I always stop using it when its efficacy for weight loss drops after several months of use.

What other side effects are related to phentermine?

Constipation, feeling jittery, and insomnia are common.

The literature shows it can raise blood pressure, and cause valvular disease and pulmonary hypertension or even death if used with dexfenfluramine (as phen-fen), which has been withdrawn from the market.

In a study, two female patients in Malaysia were reported to have heart attacks (acute myocardial infarction), possibly caused by phentermine. A study reported that a man in the US suffered from heart valve damage (aortic valve tear), possibly related to phentermine use. At the same time, a Korean study in which patients who used phentermine, were followed closely with echocardiograms or ultrasounds of the heart. It didn't show any heart valve or cardiovascular related abnormalities.

But, there is a warning regarding phentermine's cardiovascular (heart-related) side effects.

How do I know if I'm damaging my heart (cardiovascular system) while on phentermine?

These are symptoms that may indicate it is damaging your heart, including difficulty breathing, chest pain, abnormal heart sound, blood pressure, easily tired, and palpitations. If you develop any unusual symptoms while on phentermine, inform your doctor right away.

Is the damage reversible?

There were extensive researches done on the after effects of phentermine and fenfluramine (phen-fen). The studies reported that when you stop taking fenfluramine, which has been removed from the US market, the valvular abnormalities (regurgitation) return to near normal for the tricuspid and mitral valve. But this does not apply for the aortic and pulmonary valves which are also important.

So what is the verdict?

I wouldn't be afraid to take this medication for weight loss, provided the following are met:

1. BMI >30
2. Waist line of >35 for women and >40 for men
3. Short-term use (not more than six months)
4. No underlying heart disease
5. Monitored closely by a physician
6. Used together with diet and exercise
7. Awareness of warning symptoms that should be reported to a physician

By practicing medicine as a doctor, we help with our patients with difficult decisions. The basic principle for making decisions is the same, whether it's for obesity and weight loss or treatment of other medical diseases. Obesity is a disease like hypertension or diabetes or anything else.

I believe obesity is not a cosmetic issue or a personality issue. It is a medical disease. And like other medical diseases, it needs to be treated — with weight loss.

I teach my patients everyday

1. Needing a medication and not taking it is wrong. By not taking the medication, you're walking on thin ice that could crack at any time.

2. Understanding side effects prepares you to take early action if it's needed, just as though you'd move carefully on a wet surface if you saw a warning sign that it was slippery when wet.

3. Natural or herbal substances aren't necessarily safe compared to prescription drugs. We just don't know what effects they might have because they haven't been analyzed or studied systematically like prescription drugs.

Gastric bypass surgery

Among current weight loss therapies, gastric restricting surgeries are the most effective. People who go through such surgeries shed pounds massively and progressively.

Some of my patients have gone through with it, and I have several interesting chats to share with you.

After gastric bypass surgery, people receive life-changing results. Some are really good, but some are bad and can be really bad.

Here is the good stuff!

The extreme weight loss that happens can do the following:
1. It may cure diabetes.
2. It may cure sleep apnea.
3. It may cure gastroparesis.
4. It may cure cholesterol disease.
5. It may cure high blood pressure.
6. It may cure arthritis.
7. It may cure multiple infections.
8. It may result in you taking less medicines.
9. It gives you a new life with a lighter body.
10. It reclaims better health.
11. It reclaims better mobility.
12. It reclaims better breathing.
13. It reclaims better sleep.
14. It reclaims better sex.
15. It reclaims better body functions.
16. It reclaims life expectancy.
17. It reclaims social wellbeing.

It is really a life-changing, life-reclaiming surgery and treatment.

Two of my patients, Bobbie and Kathy (they are husband and wife) went through weight loss surgery; I was following them in the medical clinic.

I requested they share their stories and experience, including things that made them feel good, bad, and limited in after their surgery.

My purpose here isn't to mention what is bad about this treatment. Of course weight loss surgeries are major surgeries, with life threatening consequences at times and decision to go through such a surgery should not be taken lightly. This surgery can get us the result what we want, the big weight loss, but how we can avoid the bad effects that come with it in order to create our own weight loss without the bad effects.

1. Post-surgery, they can't eat much; they can only eat two teaspoons of liquid food at a time. One time Bobbie was eating out of the plan and he developed the dumping syndrome.

   Dumping syndrome is a complex of symptoms, including feelings of fullness, abdominal cramping or pain, nausea, vomiting, severe diarrhea, sweating, flushing, light-headedness, rapid heartbeat, hunger, confusion, fatigue, aggression, tremors, fainting, and loss of consciousness.

   Post-surgery support group attendees have all experienced the dumping syndrome, and have admitted that it's the most horrible feeling they've ever felt after the surgery, and that it's a feeling they don't want to get again.

   These symptoms are brought on by eating sugary dense foods; by consuming liquids; and by eating dairy products. Sometimes if you eat too quickly, this can also cause dumping syndrome effect post-surgery. These symptoms are bad enough that people automatically learn not to repeat their behaviors and instead strictly follow the post-surgery diet plans and portions.

2. Bobbie complained that he couldn't get enough protein in. He finally came up with the idea of putting protein powder in pill capsules and swallowing them, as he disliked the powder. He said it was terrible to eat tasteless protein in order to maintain protein requirements during the first few months.

I had to admit Kathy for dehydration and give Bobbie an infusion of fluids post-surgery, as their water and electrolyte balances were off.

So we see that there can be some undesirable effects post-surgery.

I saw Kathy and Bobbie about every few weeks, as usually one or the other had complications or suffered from side effects. But at the same time, I could also see all of their weight loss. Each week, they had visibly lost weight, and both were reaping the benefits from this weight loss.

Let's stop and think for a moment. Just because people eat less post-surgery, is that really a reason to lose weight?

Initially, you will eat about 500 calories per day before slowly increasing to 1000 calories over the course of months. This is a significant calorie deficit but it isn't the reason people lose weight, as the numbers don't match up.

Suppose a deficit of 3500 calories results in a loss of one pound of fat. You'd lose about 10 pounds per month, as the beginning of the calorie deficit might be as high as 1000 calories per day. So in two months you'd lose 20 pounds.

The weight loss post-gastric bypass surgery is much, much more. This is why the weight loss isn't because you eat less, but rather because of the transformation of the gut system that resets your weight control by changing the gastrointestinal hormones and microbes. And we have discussed this in the chapter on Ratz Stories.

From the first few days following the surgery, the transformation of these hormones and gut flora start to happen. This is very desirable change and is likely responsible for massive weight loss.

When it comes to the overweight, obese, and morbidly obese, the bigger they get, the further they get from normal weight control mechanisms, and vice versa. **The popular belief is that the bigger**

they are, the more they must be eating; this isn't true. An obese person's weight control mechanism would be out of whack, while this would be even more the case for the morbidly obese.

This is the weight control mechanism that this book is about.

The more you can keep this mechanism in stable mode, the better the weight loss and maintenance is.

Weight loss surgery resets the weight control mechanism through changes to hormones and microbiome. The weight loss effect is out of proportion to the restrictive diet post-surgery.

The resetting of the weight control mechanism through changes in stomach hormones and microbiome is thought to be due to the restrictive stomach portion effect rather than the actual surgical procedure.

The Ratz taught us this concept. Again, this popular concept-changing research is illustrated in the Ratz stories chapter.

When combined with the results of the stomach balloon inflating technique, we see encouraging weight loss when the stomach is limited in its portion.

We now know that the most reliable, effective, and safest weight control is achieved by a portion control of the stomach system.

Reduction in the absorptive surface of the gut system causes the dumping syndrome. These negative side effects are not seen with the portion control method of the weight loss.

Nutritional imbalances or vitamin deficiencies will not happen with non-surgical portion control method of weight loss.

The most important thing is to **maintain the lost weight** and stay lean; this is why we initially want to lose weight, after all. There is no point having to go through one diet after another.

Gastric bypass surgery resets the weight control system and effectively loses weight in an impressive time frame. One thing it doesn't do is to maintain the lost weight.

I had a good discussion about weight maintenance and gastric bypass surgery with a well-known bariatric surgeon.

We discussed the recurrence rate of post-bariatric surgery. In the literature, a Swedish prospective controlled study involving obese subjects showed that in five years, weight regain was 85% post-bariatric surgery.

The most likely reason for this weight re-gain is the return of the pre-surgery lifestyle and the change of the stomach hormones back to the pre-existing Fat-Me-Yes type.

Patients who underwent surgery but didn't maintain the portion control diet and healthy lifestyle wouldn't maintain the lost weight.

Some conditions when morbid obesity (or the Sick Fat) overwhelmingly overtakes the body, patients may need a drastic change like gastric surgery to reset the weight control mechanism in the body.

But mostly, obesity can be improved and maintained with the systematic portion control weight loss method and long-term lifestyle changes.

In summary, do not look for an easy way out with surgery or pills. Everything comes down to what you eat and how you eat. The Fat-Me-Not way!

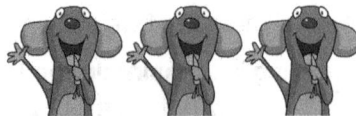

Chapter 14

Dangers Lurk in the Dieting World

Decoding Weight Loss Pills and Potions

This chapter is designed to better inform you about the pills and potions available on drugstore shelves or on the Internet. As a doctor I like my patients to be educated on these medicines and certainly would want you to know these little understood or misunderstood medicines too. Many of these weight loss medicines are available over the counter, but this doesn't make them safe. Many drugs available for weight loss are actually banned in the United States and other countries or they contain banned ingredients. Unfortunately, the Internet has made it easy for these banned drugs to be sold.

How to use this information

Whenever you see a weight-loss pill or potion, look at the list of ingredients. Often one of the following ingredients will be in it.

1. Syrup of ipecac
2. Laxatives
3. HCG
4. 2,4 DiNitrophenol
5. Guar Gum
6. Phenylpropanolamine
7. Ma Huang/Ephedra
8. Caffeine
9. Clenbuterol
10. Fenfluramine
11. Sibutramine
12. Thyroid hormone
13. Orlistat
14. Cannabinoid antagonists

Ipecac

Ipecac is an ingredient used by emergency room doctors to induce vomiting in patients who overdose on something. It causes nausea and vomiting when ingested. It also kills the appetite because of its nausea effect.

Even the 1.25mg of emetine found in ipecac is 10 times a toxic dose. Repeated use of ipecac only builds this toxicity or poisonous effect to even higher levels. So what can it do?

Ipecac causes vomiting, which can lead to aspiration and aspiration pneumonia with the vomitus going into the lungs. Severe repeated retching and vomiting could lead to tears in our food pipe (esophageal bleeding). Due to high pressure in the brain during vomiting it can even cause bleeding in the brain (intracranial hemorrhage).

But that's not all. The most dangerous effects of ipecac are on the muscles, including the heart muscles. Many people suffering from bulimia tend to use ipecac repeatedly; this results in weak and painful muscles, decreased muscle strength, heart rhythm problems, and even heart failure and cardiac arrest.

Laxatives

Laxatives have long been used to lose weight, although the science behind them is quite shaky. People suffering from bulimia are three times more likely to abuse laxatives. The problem with using laxatives is that they are not only ineffective for losing weight but can also cause many medical complications such as chronic diarrhea. Excessive laxative use causes nerve damage around the colon, leading to even more constipation problems. But the most dangerous effect of laxatives is a shifting of electrolytes in the body. This can lead to low potassium levels in the blood or low sodium levels. Since the heart is very sensitive to electrolyte levels, any such imbalance in electrolytes can lead to cardiac arrest and other heart complications.

Human Chorionic Gonadotropin (HCG)

HCG, in my opinion, is one of the biggest scams in the weight loss market. In the 1950s, it was proposed that HCG could help with weight loss when it accompanied a very low calorie diet of 500 calories a day. Later, research found that HCG does not help with weight loss; it's the very low calorie diet that causes the weight loss.

Nevertheless, HCG is also associated with low blood pressure, low sugar, constipation, and fatigue/tiredness.

Guar Gum

Guar gum is a plant fiber grown in south Asia. It is glue-like, water absorbing fibrous substance that makes you full faster and reduces fat absorption. A review of several studies done on guar gum showed no benefit for weight loss. In addition, guar gum can cause abdominal pain, bloating and gas, abdominal cramps, and diarrhea. The most dangerous side effect is obstruction of the intestines, which in some cases may even need surgery.

2,4 DiNitrophenol (DNP)

DNP is a banned substance, but it's sometimes available on the internet, sold by unscrupulous people. DNP truly speeds up the metabolism and increases fat breakdown. However, DNP is used in explosives, dyes, herbicides, and more. It can cause body temperatures to soar due to increased metabolism, and it disrupts the body's temperature control. It can cause cataracts. It can be deadly as it can also cause the heart rate to speed up, resulting in cardiac arrest.

Phenylpropanolamine

Phenylpropanolamine is a banned substance. It has been banned since 2000, but it still sometimes appears in cough syrups and diet pills. It works as a decongestant; but for weight loss, it reduces appetite. But it comes at a cost. Phenylpropanolamine can cause heart attack and brain bleeds (hemorrhagic strokes), both from excessively high blood pressure.

Ma Huang or Ephedra

Ephedra has been banned in the US since 2004, but it continues to be available in other countries and over the Internet. It is an adrenaline-boosting agent and can cause excessively high blood pressure, heart rhythm problems, heart attacks, strokes, and sudden death.

Caffeine

Take a look at the ingredients of weight loss pills, you will find many a time caffeine is used in these pills. Other ingredients, such as aspirin, can further enhance the toxic effects of caffeine. Whether caffeine causes weight loss is questionable, but it is linked to lots of side effects. Drinking coffee or other caffeine drinks and taking these pills can put you over the limit, causing nausea, vomiting, irregular heart rhythm, low potassium and calcium levels, and swelling of the brain.

Clenbuterol

Clenbuterol is used for treatment of asthma outside of the USA. Its half-life, which is a measure of how long the drug stays in our body, is more than one day. Its adrenaline-boosting effect is known to cause fat burning. But just like any medicine that boosts adrenaline, it can cause anxiety, jitters, tremors, shortness of breath, and low potassium levels. Dangerous side effects include heart rhythm problems.

Fenfluramine

Do you remember Fen-Phen®? Fenfluramine is another adrenaline-boosting drug; it was sold as a combination of Fenfluramine-Phentermine. Fenfluramine is no longer being used, though phentermine is still available, and should not be confused with Fenfluramine. Fen-Phen was removed from the market because it can cause heart valve problems. Fenfluramine, not phentermine, is also associated with increased blood pressure in the lungs, which is called primary pulmonary hypertension. Most patients with primary pulmonary hypertension die within a decade without treatment.

Sibutramine

Initially launched as a promising prescription medicine for weight loss, the FDA recalled the medicine in 2010. The weight loss effect was attributed to the medicine's ability to make you feel full while increasing the body's energy consumption. But the side effects trumped as it was linked to strokes and heart attacks.

Thyroid hormone

The thyroid hormone in the body is the driver of the metabolism. More thyroid hormone means the metabolism runs faster. If the body has less of the thyroid hormone, the metabolism runs more slowly. Too much thyroid hormone can cause weight loss by increasing the basal metabolic rate. Taking unnecessary thyroid hormone pills can lead to something called the "Thyroid Storm," a medical emergency that is as sinister as it sounds. Patients come in with high temperature, high heart rate, and tremors. Others can end up with temporary paralysis of the arms and legs, along with low potassium levels. In my practice, I have seen both.

Also chronic use of medically unnecessary higher doses of thyroid medicine can cause high output cardiac failure in which the heart is pumping so fast that it is not efficient anymore.

Orlistat

Available as an over-the-counter medicine, Orlistat inhibits the enzyme that breaks down fat in food to make it ready for absorption in the intestine. The result is that the fat doesn't break down, so it doesn't get absorbed. This causes stool incontinence, which can be embarrassing, diarrhea, and oily discharge from rectum. It can also cause deficiency in fat-soluble vitamins such as vitamin A, D, E, and K, as these vitamins get absorbed along with fat.

Rimonabant

The FDA never approved this medicine; it was withdrawn from European markets in 2009. It did reduce weight and waist circumference by blocking the cannabis-related receptors that increase appetite.

Since it has the effect opposite of cannabis, it reduces the appetite. It is associated with nausea, depression, anxiety, and tiredness.

We have now covered many of the ingredients in weight loss pills that can have dangerous side effects. This is why we shouldn't depend on these pills to lose weight. I practice what I preach. That is why in my weight loss clinic the main focus is on the diet rather than the pills. We use the SlimPlate System that designed to help lose weight without pills and powders for the same reasons above. Safety is key. There is no point losing weight only to lose your health. So always choose wisely how you are going to lose weight.

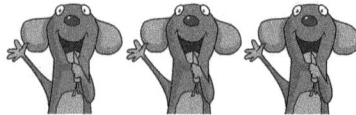

Chapter 15

Fat-Me-Not Success Strategy Part III

Fine-tuning Your Weight Loss

Do you really want to lose weight?

I told you before one of my obese patients told me that she didn't want to lose weight any longer because she had tried to lose weight several times. Every time she lost weight, she gained much more back later.

This highlights why it is so important for you to choose the right weight loss program from the start. Read this book twice if you have to but make sure you are not setting yourself up for rebound weight gain and disappointment. Her are some things you can do to start on the right foot.

💡 FAT-ME-NOT TIPS

THE DOS:

1. Choose the right weight-loss method that is biological. Don't choose it just because it sounds logical

2. Don't go for a quick fix. Even if you only have to lose ten pounds, lose it over at least eight weeks.

3. Don't eliminate out a food group completely from your diet. Don't do a no-carb diet or a no-fat diet.

4. Remember to eat more frequently, at regular intervals, but in smaller portions.

5. Be all-inclusive: include diet, exercise, support, and also medication if indicated. This point can't be stressed enough.

6. Do it easily, but persistently. Don't look for complicated solutions

7. Start your maintenance planning from the beginning, even before you start losing weight.

8. Don't start losing weight if your mental or physical health isn't stable. First get them stabilized.

9. Prevention is always the better option. Monitor your weight and start your weight loss efforts before it gets too far.

10. Don't be embarrassed to talk about your weight with your friends and family. Let them support you and do it together.

"Doctor, I don't eat much, but I'm still gaining weight. Why?"

I am frequently asked this question by my patients who have decided to go on some kind of weight-loss plan.

There are two things wrong with this question.

1. It's wrong to not eat.
2. There is something wrong with what they are eating.

Not eating regularly can make us fat.

Ideally, we should eat four-five times a day: breakfast, lunch, dinner, and snacks. Snacks can be eaten between lunch and dinner or between dinner and bedtime, depending on when you wake up and when you eat dinner.

Our brain will recognize us to be in starvation mode if we don't eat for 6-8 hours while awake. During sleep, energy expenditure drops about 10 percent, but if our bodies put us in starvation mode, energy expenditure drops by up to 40%.

What does this mean?

In starvation mode, you don't burn the calories; instead, you save them. The body saves energy as fat, especially in starvation mode. The end result is that you gain weight by accumulating fat when you don't eat regularly.

Remember! It's very important that you eat if you want to lose weight. Trying to lose weight by not eating is the totally wrong thing to do.

REBECCA

Rebecca had about twenty-two pounds of excess fat, but her body proportions looked just fine. I was surprised that she wanted to see me for weight loss. I have treated very challenging patients who weighed more than 422 pounds but it was not as difficult to treat them for weight loss, as it was to treat Rebecca.

The problem was that she was too scared to eat. She went hungry all the time and she always struggled not to eat. Whatever I told her to eat, she would reduce it by half the amount and frequency, while also doubling the amount of exercise/physical activity that I instructed her to do.

For the first few months, she struggled with what she thought was right. Finally, I had to tell her that she was doing it all wrong. Time and again, I reassured and encouraged her to try at least one month in the way that I wanted her to. She very reluctantly to start eating regularly; it took her seven months in total to lose eighteen pounds of fat, despite the fact that my 422-pound patient managed to lose seventy-eight pounds over the same amount of time.

Trust me. We were born to eat. We just need to eat in the right portions. Depriving ourselves will do us no good.

There are two types of food groups: one makes you feel satiated and full. The other makes you eat more.

Imagine yourself eating Meals A and B as follows.

Meal A: an 8 oz. glass of water, a 6 oz. grilled chicken breast, 1 cup of steamed broccoli, and 3/4 cup of cooked wild rice.

Meal B: A 16-ounce Diet Soda, a hamburger, and a medium French fries.

Lets' forget about the calorie difference between them. Just imagine how you'd feel after eating these two meals.

By eating Meal A, you'll feel full; you might feel hungry again after 4-6 hours. But you won't feel bloated, tired, fatigued, or sluggish.

By eating Meal B, you'll feel stuffy, gassy, and bloated; the initial burst of energy will be followed by sluggishness, fatigue, and a foggy mind within one hour. So you'll need to lift yourself up with another caffeine drink in a few hours; this will give you another temporary energy, ensuring that you'll need another pick-me-up chocolate or sweet treat in another few hours. You'll be busy chasing the energy burst and gain weight by drinking or eating the wrong kinds of food all day long.

How can we know what the right foods are for us? Simple! Remember to observe how you feel after what you eat. Your main drink is water, nothing else. Start by avoiding all kinds of soda, sweet tea, beer, and diet drinks.

Don't be disappointed yet. I also drink soda, but drink it the way I mentioned it in the Fat-Me-Not Success Strategy Part III Chapter.

How to eat right carbohydrates

We're always concerned about eating carbs. Carbs (glucose) are needed by every tissue of the body, especially the brain and red blood cells.

There are two kinds of carbs. Simple sugars and complex sugars (starch).

Simple sugars include sucrose, fructose, glucose, raw sugar, and molasses. It is easily digested and absorbed in the gut and raises your blood sugar quickly.

Complex sugars are starches such as potatoes, flour, vegetables, and fibers. They are also digested and absorbed in the gut, but they don't raise blood sugar as quickly as simple sugar.

How **fast** a food raises the glucose in the blood after ingesting a carb is called it's glycemic index (GI). Generally, it tells us the quality of the carbs.

The **amount** of glucose, in the particular food per serving, is called its glycemic load (GL). It also tells the quantity of the carb.

When we choose carbs, both GI and GL are important. High GI food doesn't necessarily give you high GL. It's like a marathon race. Just because you start out first, it doesn't mean that you'll finish first.

Another factor we need to consider is preparation of the food and even the age of the produce. Different potatoes, for instance, can have different GI and GL depending on preparation and the age of the produce.

It's confusing. The reason I'm explaining this concept is so you'll have correct knowledge when you read food labels.

💡 FAT-ME-NOT TIPS

I HAVE A SIMPLE PLAN FOR YOU.

1. Choose the quality of the carb by observing how you feel 1-2 hours after eating that particular carb. A high GL food will make you feel drowsy or sleepy

after eating it, while high GI foods will give you a quick feel-good, followed by feeling tired or blah after approximately 20-30 minutes.

2. **Limit** the amount of carbs that make you feel drowsy (high GL foods). **Completely avoid** carbs that only give you a quick feel-good (high GI foods).

3. If you eat prepared or prepackaged foods, check the total **sugar** content of the item. Don't eat more than than 18 grams of **sugar** every two hours. Say you want to eat chocolate chip cookies. Each cookie contains 30 grams of sugar, so eat half of the cookie now and finish the other half in two hours. The point is that you don't want to give your body a high load of sugar at a single time. Also, learn more about it in the sweet tooth section.

We have to choose the right carbs to eat. Here are some easy principles:

1. Grains: Rougher or less refined grains stay in the gut longer and provide a bigger workout for the digestive system.

2. Fruit: Fruit has good sugar, vitamins, and fiber. Eat one small fruit daily. For big fruits eat one slice only. Or if you have it, portion with the SlimPlate System's fruit saucer. You can get your own SlimPlate System from www. slimplatesystem.com

3. Vegetables: Vegetables are very low calories and rich in fiber. Make sure to eat veggies at every meal.

4. Limit sugary drinks: No soda, energy drinks, or beer Water is the best drink. But if you do consume these sugary drinks, stay **strictly** within the portion. Not more than 8 oz once a day or use the SlimPlate System cup portion. Most weight gain happens because people drink out of portion drinks, not because they eat too much.

I don't support cutting carbohydrates out completely when you're trying to lose weight.

We can eat small, frequent portions of carbs instead. Carbs not only give you energy, they also prevent you from wasting lean muscle. When you avoid carbs completely, it can reduce your weight by wasting muscle. This is because the energy now has to come from protein. Loss of muscle will reduce your metabolism and cause rebound weight gain. This is the wrong method of losing weight because it guarantees you'll gain it all back with rebound.

The cavemen didn't learn about GI or GL. They didn't count their carb intake. But obesity issues weren't as much of an issue then as they are now.

The reason we are increasingly obese is two-sided. Food makers prepare more refined and sweeter food i.e. they have both high GI and GL. As customers, we gorge on them limitlessly. I frequently see people drinking two liter bottles of soda or six cans of beer or a gallon of sweet tea or eight slices of bread, or six stacks of pancake in a single day. We've almost lost the meaning of eating. We are almost stuffing the food into our bodies.

We need to strike a balance and not be scared of eating. We were born to eat. But be careful; don't gulp a single food item in large amounts either.

How to survive in a food-abundant world

Why are we getting bigger?

Today in the United States, two out of three people are overweight. One day I sat down in a shopping mall, watching shoppers passing by. Seven out of ten people are either overweight or obese. We're so used to seeing bigger people that we forget that we might be carrying excess weight.

Once a year, I travel from Charlotte, North Carolina to Burma, in Southeast Asia, crossing either transpacific or transatlantic. As I cross through airports in different regions, I see significant differences in the people's sizes. People from America are bigger despite their different ethnicities.

So we must be doing something to make us bigger. It can't all be genetics.

So why are we different?
1. Abundant food
2. Larger portions
3. Free extras and buffets
4. Eating alone
5. Sedentary lifestyle

How do we survive in a food-abundant world?

Look at our homes and offices. We are surrounded by food: in the fridge, on the counter, in cabinets, everywhere. We lose sight of how much we eat; often we're just mindlessly munching on something. When we're stressed, we go to the fridge. When we're free, we look for something to eat. When we're bored, we keep our mouths busy. We always have plenty of food to eat. We never have to prepare, cook, or make food; it's readily available everywhere.

Due to huge market competition, restaurants and fast food places offer us extra stuff. Super-sized drinks, meal deals, buffets, abundant condiments — these are all freely available and we tend to make good use of it without realizing the excessive weight gain it brings.

When we fill up our cars with gas, we don't overfill it. But we tend to overfill ourselves with all the extras. We forget why we eat and are more interested in making good use of the abundant food.

Let's see how we can stay on course in our abundant surroundings.

In a medical clinic, we get plenty of food, sweets, and meals. When I go to the hospital, complimentary food and drinks are readily available for the physicians in the doctors' lounge. It's nice to have the food around so we don't work with an empty stomach on a busy schedule.

What do we do among all these delicious temptations when we're hungry? Ninety-nine percent of the time I'm hungry when I walk into the doctors' lounge or the break room in the clinic.

I grab a bottle of water. Then I look for fruit and nuts and gulp it down with the water. Then I choose what I want to eat to fill my stomach. Remember, smaller bites, with some pauses in between. It's very much okay not to finish a cookie in one go.

I told all of the employees at my clinic to only eat in the break room or lunchroom. Eating or drinking at your desk not only make you eat constantly but also reduces desirable physical activity. Keep candies, sweets, or chocolates in the lunchroom itself. If you want it, get up and go to the lunchroom. This gives you a bit of extra physical activity and a small break from staring at the computer screen!

When somebody brings lunch for the office, we always tell them to bring only what we really want to eat. Bringing food for twenty generic items to feed twelve people isn't a good option. Instead, each individual orders what he or she wants from the same restaurant and request them to bring just that. We don't need to eat all of the extra food.

While we are taking extra measures not to waste food, we have to remember that it's more dangerous to dump extra food into our stomachs than it is to dump it in the garbage.

At work, when you organize people into a discipline, everybody follows it because we all are in same boat. When you do it together, you're more likely to be successful. It's very okay to talk about the fact that you're watching your weight with your colleagues.

Losing weight with a sweet tooth

If you like to eat sweets or sugar dense foods, practice eating in the following manner.

Remember, sweets are not meals. You might replace a sandwich with cookies for lunch, but this isn't the right way to eat. At lunch or dinner when we need more calories, you will end up eating 5-10 cookies if you use them as meal replacement. The high sugar will keep you from burning fat; you also won't be satisfied with what you ate. Later, you'll binge-eat – remember in the Ratz Stories chapter, the rat experiment when the rat went into binge eating mode after eating sugar and fat combo. That's how behavioral problems like addiction, binging, and craving develop. Eat appropriate meals like sandwiches or pasta for meals instead of cookies or cake.

It is known that cookies and cakes both are high in sugar, and that people know not to eat them. What about eating an apple and yogurt as a meal replacement? Apples and yogurt are both healthy. What's wrong with eating these foods as a meal?

It's not a satisfying meal, and when we're not satisfied with our meals, our bodies demand more calories in different ways, like eating larger meals at a later time, food binging, and craving.

We need to eat to satisfy the stomach and the brain in order for appropriate weight control signals to be turned on in the body.

It's really important to eat real food, real sugar (not artificial sweeteners), and real meat (not protein powders or shakes) in order to satisfy our desire to eat in a normal way and maintain a normal control on weight.

You can imagine why severely obese people continue to eat constantly despite barely needing the calories. They've lost their weight control signals; their brains don't sense the satiety and so they are overwhelmed by cravings and end up binge eating.

This is true for anyone if they let themselves reach the point where they lose control.

So refuse to submit to these excuses:
- You don't have time to eat
- You can't drink water
- You must drink sugary drinks in excess
- You're addicted to diet drinks and diet sugar

Remember, even with our cars, we do regular oil changes, fill the wheels with air, align the wheels, and put in the appropriate grade of oil.

Why don't we take care of ourselves by eating healthily and at appropriate times? The further we go from eating normally, the more we derail our normal metabolism.

So refuse those bad, unhealthy habits; kick them out of your way and become healthy and lean.

I love food and enjoy eating it. I cannot stay on salad and a piece of meat. I like rice, meat, vegetables, sweets, and fruits. I like deep-fried foods and nice rich creamy coffee, too. My will power isn't very good when it comes to my food control. And I am not at all a super lean type. I'm more the kind of person who immediately shows the kinds of foods I eat in terms of weight.

So I am in the same boat as most of you.

I'll teach you how I've kept to my 127 pounds 99% of my life.

Most people trying to lose weight do have a sweet tooth.

💡 FAT-ME-NOT TIPS

The six-point plan of action for people with a sweet tooth!

1. Out of sight
2. Mix and match
3. Pause and ponder
4. Three bites principle
5. Know when to stop
6. Rescue run

OUT OF SIGHT, OUT OF MIND

Refer to the grocery shopping section coming up soon. I don't buy more than one new extra item that isn't on my shopping list when I go shopping.

Avoid getting multiple varieties of the same food. For example, if I were getting M&Ms, I wouldn't also get Hersheys, Lindt, and Godiva. Pick one at one time.

I don't keep food around long in the office or in the house if we don't plan on eating it. Extra food at home will only stimulate you to eat more, thus destroying your weight loss plan.

MIX AND MATCH

A sweet or dessert should be mixed with a different food group which can slow down sugar absorption thus decreasing its GI (Glycemic Index)

1. A level scoop of ice cream with nuts and berries
   Ice cream (protein, simple sugar), nuts (good kind of fat), berries (complex sugar)
2. Macadamia nut cookie with four ounces of milk
   (Protein, simple sugar, good fat and complex sugar)
3. A slice of whole-grain organic bread with two tablespoons of fruit jelly or peanut butter
   (Complex sugar, simple sugar, protein and fat)

The purpose of mixing food groups is to prevent the fast increase of glucose in the circulation to prevent increase in body fat due to this rapid rise of sugar and insulin. Our body absorbs different food groups (protein, fats, and carbs) at different rates.

From fastest to slowest in absorption are simple sugars, complex sugars, protein, and fat.

Mixing and matching makes us more satisfied with what we eat and also prevents us from eating all simple sugars and causing us to save fat and become fat.

PAUSE AND PONDER

We should never eat hastily, regardless of whether we're trying to lose weight or trying to maintain a healthy weight. Any meal consumption should take at least ten minutes. It is good idea to frequently put down the spoon and take a pause in between bites. Drink a few sips of water to slow down your eating. Conversation also helps. Simple things like these habits help making losing weight a long lasting one.

THREE BITES PRINCIPAL

Always remember: the first bite is for taste, the second is to confirm, and the third is for satisfaction. If you eat a chocolate truffle in one go, you'll have to eat three pieces to make you feel satisfied. If you eat one truffle in three different bites, most likely you won't need to eat three pieces. (One truffle gives you about 73 calories.) So nibble on the desserts and enjoy them, don't gobble them up. Let the desserts stay on your tongue longer. Because once the sweet taste is gone the pleasure is gone too. Avoiding extra calories is a good weight-loss plan without feeling deprived.

We always want to make sure that the food that we eat satisfies our body and mind. The longer it stays in our mouth, the faster we get satisfied.

KNOW WHEN TO STOP

When trying to maintain weight or when you're on a weight loss plan, serve food in the appropriate utensil or container. Never eat ice cream out of the tub; you'll never know when to stop. You will end up finishing the whole tub. Instead place a scoop of ice cream in a nice bowl, and decorate it with nuts and berries. When you are done eating the serving, stop.

Let's see how you should eat fresh-baked cookies if you are on a weight loss plan. Take one or two at the most out from the batch and place them on a small plate. Keep the rest in storage. Enjoy with a glass of water or a 4 oz. glass of milk. Remember the three bites principal and pause and ponder. When you are done with it, stop. Don't give yourself a chance to revisit the kitchen to see and smell the rest of the cookies.

We should also learn to stop after completion of an appropriate serving size, served in an appropriate container. Small things that we do during a weight loss plan will make your life easy as you go through the diet. Such healthy habits are also important in maintaining a healthy weight.

RESCUE RUN

There may times in our weight loss or dieting plan that we fail to follow all these measures. You eat three truffles or five cookies or half a tub of ice cream, and consequently think your weight loss plan is a disaster, that losing weight is impossible, and it feels as if someone has punched you in the stomach.

What do I do if my weight loss plan is interrupted by a binge?
Don't sit on the couch, feeling down or curl up in bed regretfully.

We have up to two hours to burn down the extra calories. If I end up gorging I quickly go in and out of the rooms in my house and pick up the laundry and start doing the dishes; I will find things to do around the house physically until I burn the extra calories down. I might even walk around the neighborhood for 30 minutes, or maybe go grocery shopping or walk around the mall. Any activity would do to salvage the weight loss plan!

If you run out of activities, as Enrique sings, sing out loud that you're tired of being sorry.

Here are some interesting facts about human eating behavior:

1. When people are given larger plates, they spontaneously eat larger portion of food.
2. Only 45% of people notice that they are eating from a larger plate.
3. Despite the size of the plate, people's satiety and hunger ratings are the same. That means you can eat from a smaller plate, smaller quantity and are satiated the same as if you were eating from a larger plate, larger quantity. We really don't need to eat a larger meal on a larger plate, but many a times we inadvertently end up doing it anyways.
4. Eating a larger meal doesn't cut down on subsequent food intake.

The more I understand about human eating behavior, the more interesting it becomes. Many of my patients told me that they didn't want to start eating as they would then eat everything without being able to control it.

Practice what we've learned here about eating sweets at your home for two months and you'll be a master at it.

Bring out one piece of dessert at a time, use small bites; with pause and ponder, you'll be surprised at how easily you feel satiated and in control.

When we eat sweets, we actually eat for the taste. As long as that satisfies us, we should be able to eat without guilt or increasing waistline. Just eat the way we learned here.

Avoiding sweets altogether isn't a good idea, as you're going to live in this healthy lifestyle for the long term. You don't want to deprive yourself of goodies for your entire life. So try eating them confidently in the ways that we learned just now.

I have put the correct portion for different sweets and chocolates in the SlimPlate mobile app so you can check to see how many pieces of chocolate you can eat at a time without feeling reluctant to eat. You can download the app for free at the Appstore or Googleplay. Just scan this QR code with your phone.

Drinks choices

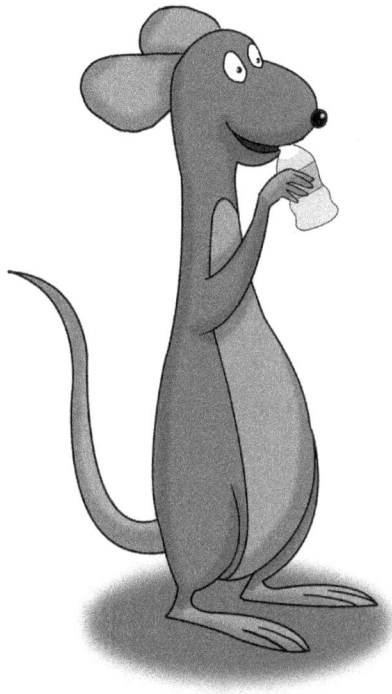

We should drink water. **Just plain, simple water**. Not flavored water. Not vitamin water. Regardless of whether or not you're on a weight-loss plan.

Drink an 8 oz. glass of water when you eat, when you feel thirsty, when you sweat, when you wake up, when you do sports, when you exercise, when you return from work/school, when you go to work/outside, when you go to bed (assuming you don't have a frequent night time urination problem).

Drink eight glasses of water a day unless restricted by a physician.

The water provides benefits, including:

1. Energy
2. Freshness
3. Flushing out waste products
4. Regulates bowel movement
5. Keeps you in neutral taste
6. Cleans mouth and oral cavity
7. Satisfies the stomach
8. Water is essential for a good weight loss program

After all, it isn't intoxicating.

SO ARE THERE ANY INTOXICATING NON-ALCOHOLIC DRINKS?

Well, we are seeing more and more evidence that drinking diet drinks in excess and regularly can harm your health. It isn't healthy to drink whether you're trying to lose weight or not.

I see in my practice that diet soda causes migraines, headaches, foggy brain, lack of energy, fatigue, palpitations, mouth ulcers, and soreness. The literature has shown even more serious conditions caused by artificial sweeteners.

Sugary drinks include regular sodas, sports drinks, and sugar-added fruit juice. Anything containing sugar in the drinks can give you excessive calories and can increase weight over time. Approximately 500 excess calories per day can add a pound of fat per week.

Have you ever looked at the total calories per serving in what you drink? One 16 oz. bottle of soda contains 200 calories. Let's say you drink one bottle a day; you'll gain one pound of fat in 2.5 weeks (17 days), approximately 20 pounds over a year.

Start looking at how many calories is in your drinks. If you like the carbonated drinks you can get carbonated water such as tonic water, or club soda.

WHAT IS BAD ABOUT EXCESSIVE AND REGULARLY DRINKING DIET AND NON-DIET SOFT DRINKS, WHEN YOU ARE TRYING TO MAINTAIN AND/OR LOSING THE WEIGHT?

1. These drinks give you extra calories making you gain weight if you drink sugary drinks.
2. Those calories are not satisfying you; instead they make you crave for more sugar.
3. Diet drinks make you eat more than you would normally eat (The research has shown that people consume up to 40% more calories when they eat after consuming a DIET drink)
4. And after the initial sugar rush and energetic feeling you will feel tired and fatigued.

SO DO I GIVE UP ON SODAS AND SUGARY DRINKS COMPLETELY?

I personally don't like diet drinks, so I don't drink them at all.

When I drink, I drink non-diet drinks.

I pour out the soda into an ice-filled 8 ounce glass. I drink this 2-3 times a week, maximum. I have something else to snack on, like wholegrain crackers, nuts, cheese, or even potato chips with soda drinks. In brief, I drink soft drinks as a special drink snack.

Yes, I gain about 75 calories from the drink and another 75 calories from the snack. When you mix simple sugars with complex sugars, protein, or fat, it prevents drastic ups and downs of sugar in the bloodstream and keeps your sugar levels steady. So it does not make you fatigued; also you don't crave more to keep up your energy.

But I don't usually quench my thirst with soda, juice, or sport drinks. My regular daily drink is just plain water.

DRINKING ALCOHOL WHILE LOSING WEIGHT

During my consultation with weight loss patients, they ask if it's all right to drink beer, wine or liquor.

Alcohol gives you 7 Cals for each gram rather than the 4 Cals of other carbs.

Alcohol is made from a carbohydrate known as barley. Before it becomes alcohol, this grain is malted to become maltose, which is then brewed to ethyl alcohol and carbon dioxide.

The **malting** process concentrates the calories, which is why alcohol gives you higher calories than other carbs.

The **brewing** process makes the alcohol chemical different from other carbs. This is why alcohol does not have a measurable glycemic index; and it doesn't break down into glucose.

So alcohol companies claim that alcohol doesn't not have much in the way of sugar, which is technically true but with a twist. We see a lot of central obesity, fatty liver, wasting of muscle, and abnormal fat deposition with regular alcohol consumption.

When you drink alcohol, it quickly absorbed into the blood stream. This is why we immediately get tipsy.

Then alcohol quickly travels through the entire body. It breaks down in the liver into acetaldehyde, then to acetyl CoA and CO_2. There is an enzyme involved in the alcohol degradation. The degree to which you feel drunk depends on this enzyme activity.

During this breakdown process, the energy residue is used up by alcohol, clogging up the body's essential energy transport system (the TCA cycle). The breakdown of glucose, fat, and the rest of the energy-yielding process are blocked until the alcohol breakdown is complete. No other nutrients get degraded until alcohol completes its degradation. This is why, when a person drinks alcohol regularly and heavily, it exhausts the body's energy transfer, which is needed for fat degradation. It causes fat deposition especially in the liver and cause fatty liver.

During the weight loss program, you desire fat burning/degradation rather than depositing/storing the fat.

So when you're trying to lose weight, you shouldn't drink alcohol in excess for at least two major reasons:

1. Alcohol isn't a nutrient, but it gives you a lot of non-nutrient calories.
2. Non-nutrient calories don't satisfy you nutritionally; you don't get full or satisfied.

Alcohol creates fat accumulation, especially central obesity; this is the opposite of what we want during weight loss.

I don't support regular alcohol use during the weight loss plan. But if you must drink, follow the portion provided in the SlimPlate mobile app. I refer you to download the mobile app because I am not able to put all these portion sizes in this book or it will become heavy and boring. Beer and various alcohol portions are listed under food suggestions. Stay within the portion provided and allow only one portion drink at a time.

Why we should cook at home

I prepare dinner in three courses. This is based on something that I learned from an old Chinese man.

When I was growing up, I had 98-year-old Chinese man as a friend. When I got up to study in the early morning, I saw this old grandpa coming back from his daily walk. Even today I can remember his face with bright eyes and smile. Even though he was nearly one hundred years old, he was walking with a straight spine and was full of energy.

His secret was very simple: Every morning, he had a glass of milk, a boiled egg, and a piece of fruit for breakfast. For lunch and dinner, he had a special soup that was made from a clear broth of water, ground garlic, salt, and pepper, with meat boiled in it. In this broth, he dips all kinds of vegetables to make them tender. I still remember how skillfully he used his chopsticks to dip vegetables into the broth and pick them back out without any tremors from old age. Then he had a small portion of meat and a small bowl of rice together.

He died at the age of 105 without suffering, losing his memory, or struggling with disease or any disabling condition. Even now, I'm amazed by how intelligent he was. He would tell me about his war experience, world history, geography, and all of his life events. He didn't need help from anybody for his daily personal care until he died. He helped his family buy groceries and keep the backyard beautiful. He was lean, healthy, and energetic despite his age.

It is very important that we take great care of our body and be careful about what we eat. I make a point to my family that we eat regularly and in a healthy way, either dining in or out. It is also very important to choose healthy snacks. Day in and day out, we are busy, and we'll always be busy. If you don't have time to take care of yourself now, you never will. So pause and think, and take some time for yourself and your family.

I make meals in thirty minutes or less. I take great pride in being able to provide healthy meals for my family. I'll share tips on how to prepare the kitchen for a daily healthy meal at your own home.

Let's buy groceries together.

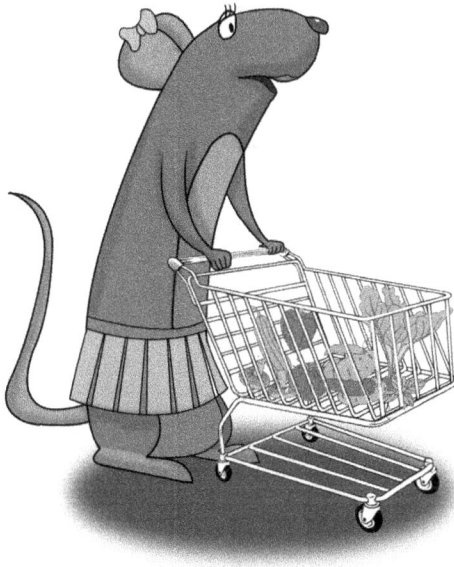

Grocery store is a place where your weight loss plan begins. It is what you buy here will decide what you eat at home. If you buy that big cake, you will have no choice but to eat it when you get home. So you have to start making choices at the grocery store, not at home.

☀ FAT-ME-NOT TIPS

LET ME TELL YOU HOW TO BUY GROCERIES:

1. Keep a checklist on your fridge of what you need to buy for your family.

2. Organize basic items needed in a typical week, like bread, eggs, milk, orange juice, etc.

3. Choose the healthier versions of the basic items your family eats frequently.

4. Snacks: Choose nuts, berries, fruit, and snacks you prepare yourself, or potato or tortilla chips.

5. Pastries and bakeries: Most snacks from store shelves contain unhealthy fat and should be avoided. It's better to have freshly prepared cookies than cookies from the shelf.

6. Greens and vegetables: Shop for a lot of vegetables, such as spinach, broccoli, and assorted colorful peppers. The more color you can include, the better it is.

7. Meat: Shop for lean-cut meat of any kind. Avoid processed and ground meat. If you need ground meat, buy a grinder, or ask the butcher to grind your lean cut separately. Never buy the commercially available ground meat, as it has double the amount of fat.

8. Seafood: Buy abundant amounts of fish, shrimp, and prawns. Buy only fish caught in the wild. Farm-raised fish aren't a good option even though they're cheaper; they won't have good omega 3

fatty acids compared to wild-caught fish. In farms, fish don't get a healthy diet, so they aren't free from antibiotics or GMOs.

9. Drinks: Plain, simple water. Your main drink needs to be water. If you ask me what the biggest root cause of obesity is, I'd have to say that it's drinking sugary drinks.

10. Juice: Juice isn't a bad thing, but be careful of serving size and type. Buy juice that doesn't have added sugar to it.

11. Munchies/boredom food: You can eat various snacks off the shelf, but you can also create something that will be your own fancy snack. This will entertain you at night and will also mean you engage in some physical activity. Make sure you mix complex sugars and protein in your snacks as we discussed before.

12. Don't buy food items just because they're on sale.

13. Don't shop when you're hungry unless you have your shopping list and you know you're going to stick to it.

14. Don't buy more than one extra item not on your list.

You may feel you healthy foods are not tasty. When we change our food habits, the taste buds in the tongue also adapt to the change fairly quickly. Try it to believe it!

💡 FAT-ME-NOT TIPS

HERE IS THE HEALTHY VERSION OF DAILY FOOD ITEMS!

1. Lean-cut meat, regardless of whether it's beef, pork, turkey, or chicken

2. 2% or skim milk

3. Low-fat cheese and dairy products

4. Whole grains, regardless of whether it's wheat, barley, oats, or rye

5. Avoid/Limit processed meats like bacon and sausage

6. Don't buy sugary drinks or soda in bulk; instead buy them occasionally from vending machines. Calories are more expensive than the cost over the long run.

7. Only buy pastries and items from bakeries as you'll eat them the same day; never buy more pieces than the members in the family.

8. Buy no sugar-added juice

9. Buy no-cholesterol oil (check the label)

10. Buy regular, organic eggs (not egg beaters)

11. Buy plenty of ginger, garlic, and onions

12. Buy plenty of lentils/pulses

13. Don't buy cigarettes

It is very important to buy groceries using a list. Stick with the list. Don't buy items because they're on sale. If the item is good and it's on your list and it's on sale, that's fine. But don't change good, nutritious, healthy food for non-healthy food that's a few dollars cheaper.

I wish we had a robot to buy our groceries so that sale tactics couldn't persuade us. Stick to your list. Pretend you're a robot when you shop for groceries.

Let's get kitchen ready to lose weight!

I never had a formal training in the culinary arts, nor am I a chef. I get nervous if I have to prepare a meal for a large crowd.

Based on my knowledge of nutrition, physiology, and medicine, I believe I cook healthy, nutritious, and simple meals for my family.

💡 FAT-ME-NOT TIPS

HERE ARE SOME TIPS THAT I SHARE WITH MY PATIENTS.

1. Get into the habit of preparing meals at home.
2. If you eat out, you lose control of portions, ingredients, money, and you also lose the fun of eating at home with your family.
3. Prepare meals fresh every day. Cooking is an exercise too!
4. Buy healthy versions of items.
5. Prepare your kitchen with the plan for success.

Plan for success

Success always starts with a plan.

Contingency is always part of the plan to success.

It's hard to prepare meals daily when you don't prepare in advance. This is how I prepare for it.

I do my major grocery shopping once a month. The same day, I divide the meat in appropriate portions in containers before freezing it.

Cut, clean, wash, drain out water (as appropriate), and keep them in reusable containers for the each meal. If you have family of four, keep the packages made for four, no more than that. You do not store them as you bought from the store. Then it will lead to waste or excessive portion consumption.

If you buy a tray of twenty pieces of chicken breast, and you have family of four, resize them in five containers with four pieces in each container. This way you don't have a chance of cooking more than what your portions should be. The portion control starts now.

The same is true for vegetables. Resize them in a zip lock bag with a portion that is appropriate for your family. For example, you have a regular size cauliflower bunch and you are preparing for two people, cut it in half. Keep each half in a zip lock bag for each meal, and then store them in the fridge or freezer. This will keep them fresh if you do that when you buy them.

I prepare the major cooking condiments every two weeks.

Peel the garlic, ginger, and the onion. I have two separate containers for each of them. One is for use in the first week, to keep in refrigerator, and one for the second week, to keep in the freezer. When you finish the first container, transfer the second container from the freezer to the refrigerator.

I suggest using plenty of the above three as appropriate. They not only enhance the flavor of the meal, but they're healthy ingredients.

The other ingredient that I use a lot in the preparation of meat and fish is the **yellow powder (turmeric powder)**. This is widely used in Indian, Malaysian, Indonesian, and Chinese cuisine. It takes away the smell of raw fish and meat and doesn't alter the taste. Most importantly, it has multiple health benefits, including anti-inflammatory and digestive effects.

Most of my cooking is done with garlic, ginger, onion, turmeric powder, salt, and chili powder.

Sometime I use saffron, cinnamon sticks, basil leaves, coriander seeds, cumin seeds, bay leaves, mint, cilantro and soy sauce.

I never use butter, ghee, margarine, or alcohol in my cooking.

So now your kitchen is ready for cooking simple daily meals.

Why we should avoid cooking with butter

Fat belongs to a calorie-dense food group. One gram of fat gives 9 calories, while protein and carbohydrates only gives 4 calories.

Worse than the high calories is the saturated fat and cholesterol content in butter. Olive oil is also calorie-dense but contains less saturated fat and no cholesterol. Cooking and eating a meal is an everyday thing. If we eat a buttered meal every day, we turn our circulatory system (arteries) into buttered arteries.

Blocked arteries are arteries filled with cholesterol and blood clots.

If you find a blocked artery in one area of your body, that means you have a high chance of having multiple arteries blocked in different parts of the body. For example, if you have blocked arteries in your heart, you are likely to have blocked arteries in your brain, in the carotid (large neck) arteries, leg arteries, arteries going into the kidneys, and the retinal (eye) arteries.

What can we do about it? How can we prevent it?

Simple! Don't regularly consume foods high in saturated fat such as butter, cheese, cream and animal fat.

Here are the devils to our arteries and to our health.

Cheese

Generally, all kinds of cheese have high saturated fat and cholesterol content, with the exception of mozzarella, ricotta, and cottage
cheese. Do look at the food label for details, as different preparations
can change the individual content. Make sure you choose low fat or
no fat versions of mozzarella, ricotta, and cottage cheese.

Butter

Generally, all butter is high in saturated fat. You can use "I can't
believe it's not butter". Again, use sparingly as it does still have high
calories, or use butter spray.

Cream

Whipped cream and sour cream are calorie-rich extra toppings.
Use sparingly. Heavy cream and half and half are high cholesterol,
artery-clogging devils. Stay away from them.

How can you control your use of butter?

Fat is calorie-dense; one tablespoonful of oil or butter will give
you 120 calories on average.

This is like one and half pieces of toast or one and half eggs, so
you can see how a single tablespoon of butter contains the same
number of calories as these foods.

So I advise you to use oil/butter spray as it has far fewer calories
and you still can enjoy the flavor of butter and olive oil.

There isn't much calorie difference between good and bad fat.
But bad fat sticks to the arteries and causes heart attacks and
strokes. So clearly it isn't good to use at your home. This practice is
more to do with good health rather than losing weight.

Cooking with butter doesn't taste better, either. Say no to cooking with butter for clean arteries. Replace your cooking base with olive or canola oil.

What to drink during the weight loss phase

Here are some non-calorie or low calories drink suggestions for when you're on the weight loss plan.

Obviously, sweet (or sugar loaded) drinks give you non-nutritive calories, which work against your weight loss plan. Multiple studies have shown that daily regular drinking of sweetened drinks can negatively alter your metabolism. In the long run, it can increase the chance of developing glucose intolerance (also called pre-diabetes), diabetes, and can even cause metabolic syndrome.

So can we turn to diet drinks? Diet drinks are sweetened with artificial sweeteners. Saccharin, aspartame, sucralose, neotame, and acesulfame potassium are used to sweeten the taste without adding calories. Diet drinks are not a better alternative to non-diet drinks. Diet drinks may make you eat more calories even though it doesn't contain any calories by itself. Artificial sweeteners may also increase your health risks if you consume them regularly.

So what we can drink when we are trying to lose weight?

You can safely drink water, lots of water, during weight loss.

FAT-ME-NOT TIPS

WHAT IF YOU'RE NOT A WATER PERSON OR JUST SIMPLY LIKE TO HAVE ALTERNATIVES?

1. Different varieties of hot and cold green tea are an alternative. Don't put sugar or sweeteners in it.

I personally find that a nice cup of hot green tea is like a tasty glass of wine. It makes me feel warm, relaxed, and pampered. I drink several cups of green tea throughout the day. It doesn't give me the high and low of sugar, no calories, or the feeling of being intoxicated. Research has shown multiple health benefits related to green tea.

Don't put sugar in it. You'll get used to its mild bitter taste like you get used to wine, without dealing with intoxicating effects.

2. My other favorite drink is lemon water.

Once a week, I peel a few lemons and puree it; it can be stored in the fridge for almost a week. At dinner, mix two spoons of lemon puree with a jug of cool water and add a pinch of salt. A few very thinly cut pieces of lemon peel may give you an augmented digestive effect for the meal you've just eaten. It's refreshing and flavorful and not fattening.

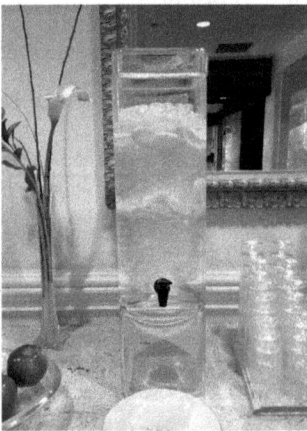

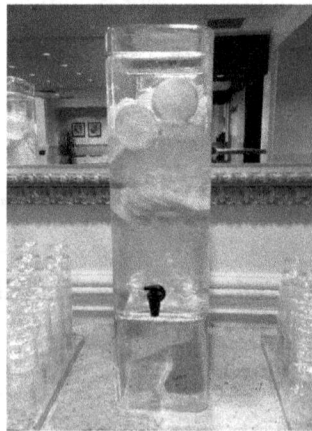

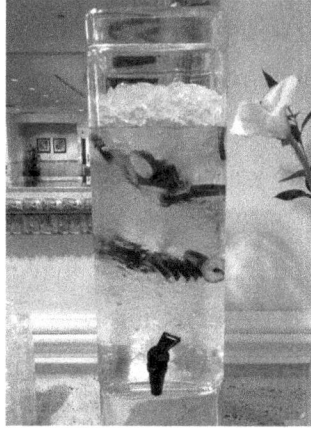

3. Fruit water/antioxidant drinks

   You can create pretty much any kind of flavored water with your favorite fruits. All fruits have fructose sugar in it, so it'll give you some calories. Roughly one cup of low calorie-yielding fruit will give you about 30-50 calories. Low calorie-yielding fruit includes watermelon, papaya, cherries, pears, apples, oranges, peaches, berries (blueberries give more calories than strawberries or raspberries). Bananas, mangoes, and honeydew are higher in calories (100-200). Grapes and grapefruit are around 60-70 calories.

   Fruit waters I like include coconut water (not coconut milk), cucumber water, and watermelon water.

   The preparation is simple. Blend a cup of cut watermelon, ice, and water into a thin drink. Chop some mint leaves and add a pinch of salt.

You can create fruit water at dinner at every night. They are fresh, give you healthy antioxidants, and a small number of calories. But remember to portion each drink appropriately.

If you must sweeten your drink, add a level teaspoon of sugar to your cup.

Some of my patients have asked if they can get commercially prepared drinks labeled as fruit water.

My answer to that is I prefer that you prepare it yourself. It doesn't take time to prepare and it's fun. It's in your control. You'll be proud that you are health cautious and that you care about yourself and your family. It will become a tradition for your family members to gather around the table for dinner and that will be your traditional drink. It will build good memories for your kids. Preparing the meal or drinks will burn some calories, too. Most of all, you will have control over the ingredients in your drinks.

The biggest issue with commercially prepared drinks, whether they're diet or non-diet, is that you lose your control over the portion and the ingredients used to prepare the drinks for longer shelf life. Also you are unlikely to leave half of the can or bottle of soda for the next time. So you are forced to finish the whole container.

Handling the party while losing weight

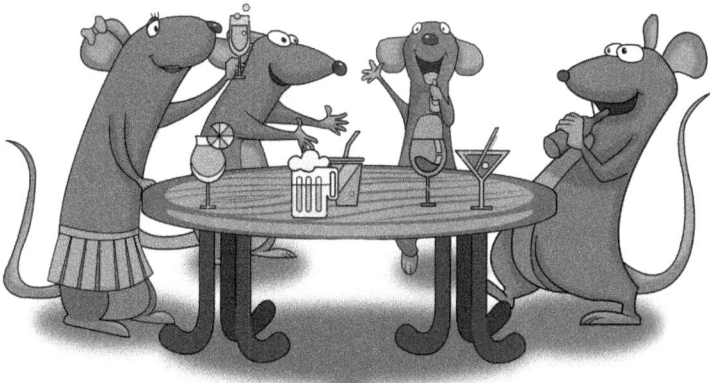

Parties are for mingling, socializing, making small talk, having a good time, and making memories.

It should **not** be an excuse for gaining weight.

Often, common knowledge just passes by in our busy mind until we acknowledge it. But once you acknowledge it, it stays with you. It's that simple.

I'm a focused person, and when I'm working on something, I forget my surroundings. I don't like that habit; I acknowledge that I even forget to smile or make a small talk with my colleagues. So one day I realized that I needed to improve this. I made a point of smiling and greeting or talking with anyone who passed by. That's it. It needs a switch and once the switch is on, everything else becomes spontaneous.

So let us turn on the switch and acknowledge that parties are for mingling and socializing, but are not an excuse to gain weight. You will realize eating won't be the priority at the parties anymore.

But the party food will test our will. Unfortunately we do not have super willpower, so we have to plan to succeed in this.

Here is our action plan for weight loss during party time!

1. Have a snack prior to going to the party so you won't arrive starving. The best is 10 nuts, a few pieces of chopped avocado, or a boiled egg. They contain good fat and it stimulates the CCK hormone in our gut, which enhances satiety so we don't overeat.

2. Start with the less dense/lower calorie foods in small portions.
   Choose less calorie dense food. The idea is not to eat high calorie-dense food when you're starving as you may eat too much. Shrimp cocktails are a more calorie-friendly choice than cheese-filled crab cakes. It is not that we're going to avoid crab cake completely, but we're going to keep it for the last. That way we don't end up eating five pieces of it and feel regretful for eating too much.
   That's the idea. Choose lean protein over cheesy and fatty foods.

3. Drink a glass of ice water.
   Always feel free to pick up a glass of water at any time: before eating, in between eating, after eating. Then if you like other drinks, you can have them in controlled portions. Let's say that you reach the party and someone offers you a drink. You ask for a glass of water first so that your thirst is quenched. Then you drink a special drink like a soft drink or

even a hard drink; you'll be drinking it for pleasure, not for thirst. We don't want to drink calories for thirst. We want to drink calories for taste and pleasure. Make this a habit, drink anything after drinking a glass of water so that you know you aren't gulping down the calories for thirst.

4. Don't sit in one place; walk around to stay connected with other people.
Engage in conversation, make connections, and get interested in others. Life is full of other things and other interests; this is the best time to get to know all these.
I like parties for that reason; I can talk about myself a little and then learn from others what they have been up to. People are happy at parties, with uplifting attire and cheerful discussions; even boastful talks are fun and interesting.

5. Take the smallest portions of cakes and sweets. Generally, two fingers width piece of cake is okay to eat. How we will savor and eat sweets is already been covered in the sweet tooth section.

6. Limit alcohol intake. This is how you portion popular drinks so that you can drink enough to enjoy and feel flushed but not increase your waistline. Ultimately, we just want to have fun without losing our guard and girth.

Keep your weight loss while travelling

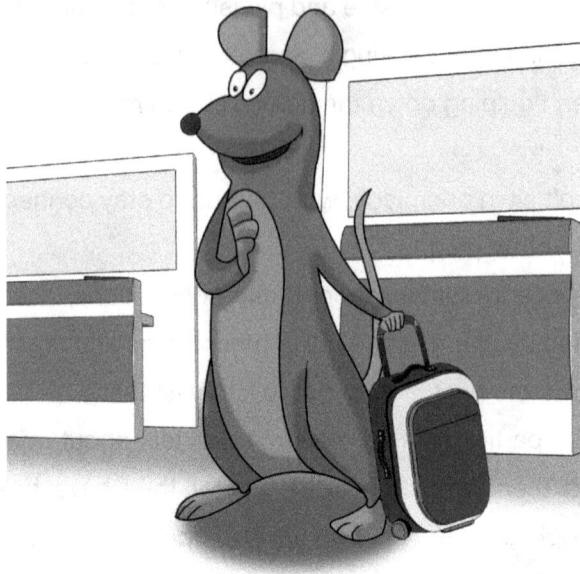

My patients often tell me that they travel a lot due to their jobs, and that they gain a lot of weight while traveling.

Let's see how we can turn this to our advantage.

Here is our action plan for weight loss during travelling.

1. Hydration is key when traveling.

   Before you check into a hotel, stock up with water from a nearby convenience store so you don't end up buying expensive water in the hotel or staying dehydrated.

2. Check out the organization's gym. I always like to see what facilities they have and put my hands on something new. Be curious, be young. You can either sit in bed

watching TV or you can work out while you watch TV. Make the right call.

3. Keep 100-calories snacks in your bag so that you can keep your metabolism up throughout the day.
   Eat small, frequent meals and don't let yourself feel like you're starving.

4. As always, portion control is key.
   You might be eating different kinds of food, but the important thing is to keep your portions in check.

Keep your weight loss while eating out at a restaurant

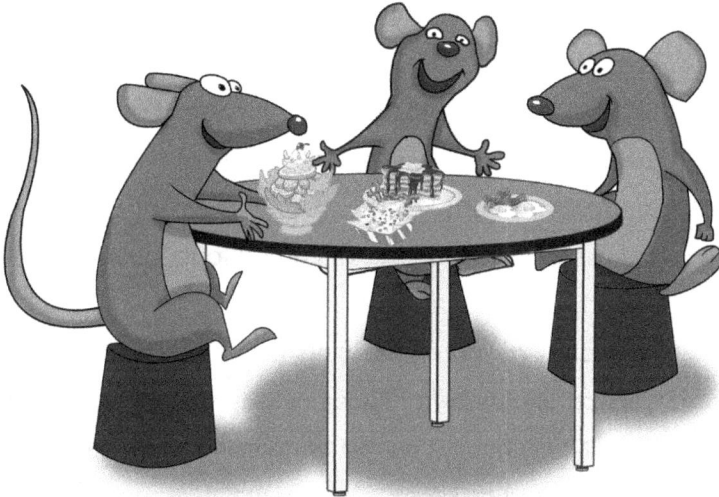

Eating out is another common practice that we do. Generally, restaurant food is rich in calories and is two or three times the calories you need for your meal.

If you are eating out for convenience, for fun, or for work-related functions 2-3 times per week, your chances of gaining weight are higher.

Fast food and fine dining restaurants both have high fat and high calorie meals. More expensive food doesn't mean it is healthier; so don't fall into that trap.

Here is the action plan for weight loss while eating at a restaurant.

1. Order one appetizer and one entrée for two people to share, if you're eating with someone. If this isn't convenient, put at least half of the food in a to-go box.
2. Skip the appetizer if possible and go straight to the entrée.
3. Ask for water and drink it first. Then only order other drinks, as often you'll realize that you don't need other drinks.
4. Avoid all-you-can-eat buffets at all costs. Food may be cheap but it's your health at stake.
5. Say no to desserts.
6. Say yes to grilled, boiled, or curried food, but no to deep-fried food with bread crumbles.
7. Always ask for gravy, dressing, and sauce on the side. A spoonful of gravy or sauce usually has 100 calories or more. Consuming a packet of dressing is like eating a slice of bread or a 2 oz. piece of meat. We need to limit these hidden calories

So do we have to stay away from it completely? No. I always ask for gravy and sauce on the side, and then use it as a dip. You don't have to eat all the gravy.

If I were to go to Steakhouse, I'd cut a thin slice of meat and dip it into the gravy just a bit, rather than pour all of the gravy onto the plate. All I want from the gravy is the flavor, not the oily taste on my tongue.

I do eat out often, for many reasons. The most important thing is to enjoy the moment with the people you're with, whatever the reason might be.

I skip most fancy drinks; my favorite drink is usually water. Sharing an appetizer and an entrée with my husband is something that I commonly do. Even if you overeat, you still can use your energy by walking around the neighborhood for an extra 15 minutes. This will make you feel better physically and mentally, and you'll always enjoy a relaxing walk anyway.

Every year for about 10 years now, I've gone around the world, and as I've passed through different airports, experiencing different foods. I've also seen many different people with different sizes in different countries.

I'm curious about what others are eating and what their sizes are.

My observation is that it is not the types of food we eat, but the portions we eat, that result in our sizes.

South East Asians, such as Japanese and Koreans, eat rice, seafood, meat, and vegetables and have a 3 to 4% obesity rate.

Mediterranean eat a good mix of starch (rice or bread or pita), lean meat, and vegetables. They have very low obesity rate, too.

Mexican food is a good mix of starch (rice/bread), beans, vegetables, and meat. But they have the highest obesity rate.

Most developed countries like America, the UK, and Australia have adopted high fat diets and much larger portions. And have one of the highest obesity rates.

Pizza from Italy and pizza from the United States are not the same. Pizza in the United States is much higher in fat, much larger in size, thicker and has humongous amounts of cheese on it as compared to a pizza made in a traditional Italian home.

The point is that foods like pizza and French fries aren't bad foods.

Similarly, if you compare Fried Chicken from United States and from Singapore, portion sizes are much different. I can share the food plate here in the United States with my husband but I can't share the same in Singapore, because the portion size in Singapore is just enough for one person.

I can share coffee here in United States with my husband, but I can't do that in Italy. The coffee portion in Italy is just for one person. In the United States, the portion is generally for two people or more.

Handling nighttime cravings like a pro while trying to lose weight

We often like to keep eating in the evening, one item after another. TV ads call out food; seems like during the day you were busy and evenings are the time to eat through the night.

Sometimes we just go to the fridge for something to put in our mouths, just wanting something to munch on.

This is how we can eat a lot of calories without realizing it.

Schedule purposeful, non-food related projects every night. For example: laundry night, Saturday Night Live old episodes review night, movie night, book club night, homework night, dance-off night, Facebook night, or anything else that makes your evening fun and purposeful.

Sometime we stay up late and need to eat a snack. This is perfectly okay; just eat at the dinner table, using right portions (the fruit saucer for SlimPlate users) so you're not mindlessly eating calories. Always have a cup of water with you.

Brush your teeth after dinner; this helps many patients who struggle to control night time eating.

Eat a mint, like a tic-tac or a small, sugarless mint.

I don't expect my patients to have super willpower as they try to lose weight. So here are the tips how you can avoid temptations.

💡 FAT-ME-NOT TIPS

Prevent unnecessary calorie intake by:

1. Avoiding grocery shopping when you're hungry so you don't end up buying the entire store and can stick to your list.
2. Avoiding surrounding yourself with food.
3. Not keeping food out on tables or counters. Food must be in the fridge or pantry.
4. Keeping food in the break room at the office so that it's not readily visible on your desk.

Portion control is key

It's not about eating; it's about eating the right amounts.

Portions are the key for losing weight and keeping it off.

I created this Fat-Me-Not weight loss plan. I know about weight loss and how to help others, but I still use the SlimPlate system every time I eat so I do not deviate. Similarly you have to be vigilant about your food portions and balanced diet.

Why? We are human beings, and what we know sometimes differs from what we practice. At dinner, I'm just a very hungry woman who sits down at the dinner table after a long day of work. Without SlimPlate System, I would be overeating 90% of the time and I'd be gaining weight like everyone else.

SlimPlate System controls what you eat and how much you eat without making you realize it. That is the beauty of it. I often may get lazy or forget to add vegetables or protein in my diet if I don't use SlimPlate. But with SlimPlate, I don't have to think. It's a visual reminder to eat a well-balanced meal at every time. That is the key to healthy weight loss. It should be easy and spontaneous.

Many people who know me personally, remark on how I stay busy throughout the day. Being busy and keeping ourselves healthy must go hand-in-hand; it cannot be only one or the other.

The main reason I am able to stay energetic despite being very busy is that I eat very regularly. I eat five times a day. That is what I advise in this book too.

So eat regularly and stay hydrated; don't skip meals. Eating less isn't the solution for losing weight; eating right is.

How to eat deep fried food and still lose weight

I eat deep-fried food at least four times a week.

You might think that weight loss and deep-fried foods don't work together.

You can deep fry meat and seafood without coating them in batter paste.

As an example, here's fried chicken and fried beef cubes.

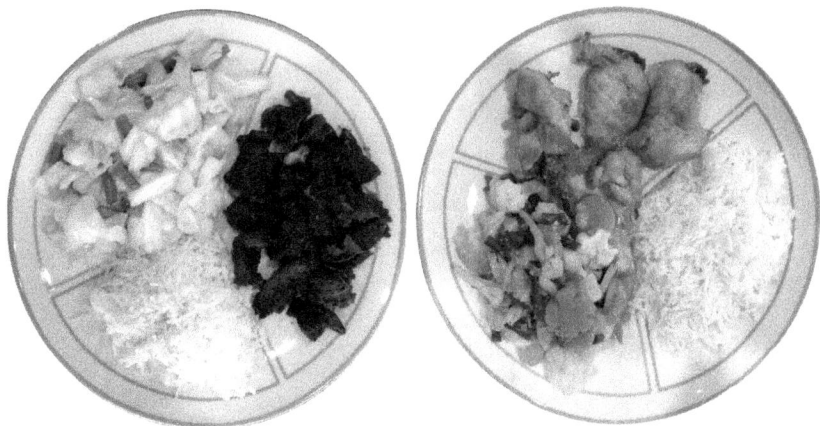

I did a little experiment at my kitchen. I poured out a cup of vegetable oil and fried a whole chicken in pieces, as shown in the picture. Without using a batter paste, I marinated the chicken with ginger and salt and fried it in hot oil.

I measure the leftover oil when I was done; it was only one and half spoons less than a cup. Basically, one and half spoons went into the fried chicken, which isn't much. It comes to about 200 calories from deep fry, divided by seven family members.

It's really not a big deal.

I like fried food, so I fry fish, shrimp, beef, and chicken. The key here is not coating the meat with batter paste. Because it is the batter paste that absorbs the most oil.

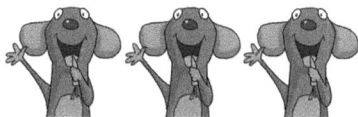

Chapter 16

Fat-Me-Not Success Strategy Part IV

Exercising to Enhance Weight Loss

You might think, as I've written about how diet trumps exercise, that exercise or physical activity isn't needed for weight loss.

Exercise and physical activity are two of the big keys to losing weight. But we need to have the facts clear and understand what to expect from exercise.

Often, my patients come and tell me that they've walked every day for six months, but haven't lost their excess weight. And they get discouraged.

Or they come to me and explain that they can't walk because of a bad knee, and feel hopeless about losing weight. It seems like weight loss is not possible anymore.

Doing half an hour or an hour of exercise won't help you lose enough weight. But it helps you in many other ways with ongoing weight-loss, provided you combine it with a balanced diet.

I'm not talking about professional athletic-like exercise or strenuous exercise. I am talking about regular people who go to the gym for an hour, or go out for a walk or go swimming.

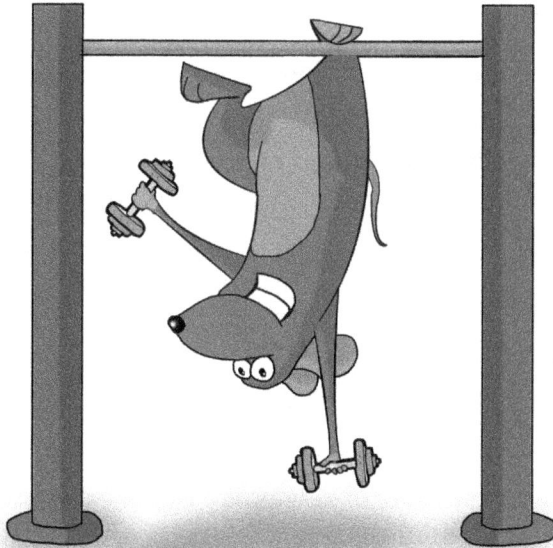

There are many benefits to regular exercise, including:

1. Maintaining reduced body weight/fat
2. Preventing weight gain
3. Decreasing blood pressure
4. Decreasing bad cholesterol and increasing good cholesterol (maintaining a good heart and brain)
5. Keeping diabetes in control
6. Decreasing the risk of cancer
7. Preventing osteoporosis and ensuring bone strength
8. Increasing cardiac output and improving endurance and stamina
9. Decreasing stress, anxiety, and depression
10. Maintaining lean body mass
11. Improving lung capacity
12. Reducing the risk of heart attack

13. Reducing the risk of stroke
14. Improving immunity
15. Keeping you healthy and looking young!

Exercise also offers weight-loss benefits, including:
1. Promoting metabolism and burning additional calories
2. Building muscle strength and helping reduce the risk of regaining weight
3. Improving stamina
4. Improving sense of well-being
5. Improving stress control
6. Improving control of depression and anxiety
7. Improving sleep
8. Improving bone strength

HOW DO YOU CHOOSE GOOD EXERCISE?

Exercise should be done every day, and an exercise plan should be created to suit each individual.

Think what kind of exercise will make you stick to it every day. Don't pick painful, strenuous exercise that you aren't going to want to do every day for the rest of your life.

I don't want you to choose an intimidating exercise that will scare you away from exercising forever. The truth is that you don't have to do strenuous exercise to lose weight, either. You're not missing out on much if you can't do, or don't want to do, strenuous exercise.

In our daily lives, we have enough things to do, so think of something that will make you smile and be happy. Just pick that one thing and incorporate it in your exercise.

I like to listen to music; it makes me feel young and free. I don't like to run, but I do like to twist.

So I choose to dance!

Start from that point. The goal is to develop a habit of doing something that you like as activity or exercise. Then once you're hooked on doing your favorite activity, you can add and modify as you progress.

You already have flexibility and stamina from doing regular exercise; you can play sports like tennis or racket ball or swimming, as it's feasible around your life.

My daily workout is dancing and hula hooping, but I sometimes play tennis, racket ball, and golf, or go swimming.

Put it this way, exercise doesn't seem at all scary.

Don't expect that doing daily exercise means you will lose ten pounds in three months. You won't lose weight just from exercising. But when you combine it with a balanced diet, rest assured that you're on your way to shaping up.

Burn More Calories: 10 Great Tips to Increase Physical Activity

There are three ways to burn more calories effortlessly.

1. Increase physical activity
2. Increase thermogenic effect
3. Increase strength

Most people who need to increase their physical activity don't have time to spend hours at the gym.

I want to suggest some small things that will help you burn calories without needing to drastically change your routine.

💡 FAT-ME-NOT TIPS

Here are ten easy tricks to help you kick off extra calories semi-effortlessly. Remember that frequent small activities can make you thin, too!

1. Pace while talking on the phone.
2. Get up and talk to people at the office rather than using email or an intercom.
3. Get up every time an ad comes on TV.
4. Dance to any music you hear.
5. Start a garden in your backyard.
6. Go shopping frequently (walking around window-shopping helps burn calories without spending).
7. While shopping, try on clothes to see if they fit; looking at yourself in the mirror should be fun and energizing, and the extra movement burns more calories.
8. Take a walk and just think. This is my favorite; I call it my thinking trail.
9. Tap and fidget whenever you like.
10. When you do chores, keep the music on. Sing aloud and dance whenever you can — make the kitchen as your own stage.

Burn More Calories: Boost Your Thermogenic Effect

The themogenic effect is the amount of body heat produced by any food. The more body heat you generate, the more calories your body burns, boosting your metabolism.

FAT-ME-NOT TIPS

5 TIPS TO INCREASE YOUR THERMOGENIC EFFECT

1. Drink a hot cup of black coffee.
2. Eat spicy food.
3. Eat something chewy; this makes your gut system work harder. Stick with low-calorie foods like celery or gum. Some candy is chewy, but because of the high calories you'll end up consuming more calories than you burn. Did you know celery has no calories? This means that chewing and digesting celery results in negative calories.
4. Eat real food rather than processed or pre-packaged bars or shakes. This can promote thermic effect by 50%, as it burns fat more effectively.
5. Eat hot food.

Burn More Calories: Increase Your Strength

Try small movements to increase strength and flexibility. If you can't do them yet, don't give up. Keep trying every day, and one day you'll get there.

1. Touch your chin to your chest.
2. Touch your fingertips to your toes, bending from the waist.
3. Clasp your hands in front, stretching your arms.
4. Clasp your hands behind your back.
5. Clasp your hands above your head.

Increase your endurance by increasing the distance you walk each day. Even if you can only walk a small block, do that every day. Before you know it, it becomes a breeze. If you need a guide from a fitness trainer, download the SlimPlate app (for Android and iPhone) and you can get various levels of exercise videos. The app is free to download; you can do these exercises at home at your convenience with no expensive equipment. No excuses!

Success means better health! Reward yourself with this positive achievement.

Warm Up

Wram up for five minutes using any combination of the four warm up videos(1 rep of 10)

• Good Morning with Dowel	• Toy Soldiers
• First Shoulder Pass Thru	• March in Place

Workout

Work out for 15-18 minutes using any combination of exercise videos at your fitness level (2 reps of 10):

Beginner:	Intermediate:	Advanced:
• Wall Push-Up	• Jumping Jacks	• Double Toe Taps
• Heel Kick w/ Band	• Ab Crunch w/ Stability Ball	• Bosu Trunk Twist
• Body Weight Chair Squats	• Squat Press w/ Band	• Kick Out on Bosu
• Knee Lift with Medicine Ball	• Skipping Rope	• Medicine Ball Lunge
• Quadruplex	• Mountain Climber on Bench	• Burbees
• Leg Drop w/ Bent Knee	**Intermediate 2:**	• Toe Touch w/ Press
	• Kettle Bell Swing	
	• Step Up	
	• Cross Over Push-Up	
	• Thrusters	
	• T-Plank Rotation	
	• Medicine Ball Slam	

Challenge

Choose a challenge for your current fitness level (2 reps of 10):

Challenge 1:	Challenge 2:	Challenge 3:
• 5 Box Jumps	• Hand Release Push-Up	• Kettle Bell Deadlift
• 10 Thrusters	• Kettle Bell Swing	• Burpee
• 10 Burpees	• Kettle Bell Deadlift	

Stretch

Choose a stretching exercise (2 reps of 10):

• Sun Salutation	• Cat Cow Stretch
• Downward Dog	• Thread the Needle
• Runners Lunge	• Hamstring Stretch w/ Band
• Child Pose	• Crossover Stretch
• Stretching Altogether	

References:

- **Glucose uptake by the brain on chronic high-protein weight-loss diets with either moderate or low amounts of carbohydrate.** Br J Nutr. 2014 Feb ;111(4):586-97. doi: 10.1017/S0007114513002900.
- **Obesity as malnutrition: the role of capitalism in the obesity global epidemic.** Am J Hum Biol. 2012 May-Jun ;24(3):261-76. doi: 10.1002/ajhb.22253. Epub 2012 Mar 2.
- **Shift work: health, performance and safety problems, traditional countermeasures, and innovative management strategies to reduce circadian misalignment** Nature and Science of Sleep. 2012; 4()111
- **Obesity alters gut microbial ecology.** Proc Natl Acad Sci U S A. 2005 Aug 2 ;102(31):11070-5. Epub 2005 Jul 20 .
- **Drug-induced weight gain.** Drugs Today (Barc). 2005 Aug ;41(8):547-55.
- **Alogliptin improves steroid-induced hyperglycemia in treatment-naïve Japanese patients with chronic kidney disease by decrease of plasma glucagon levels** Medical Science Monitor : International Medical Journal of Experimental and Clinical Research. 2014; 20()587
- **Alogliptin improves steroid-induced hyperglycemia in treatment-naïve Japanese patients with chronic kidney disease by decrease of plasma glucagon levels.** Med Sci Monit. 2014 Apr 10 ;20:587-93. doi: 10.12659/MSM.889872.
- **2013 AHA/ACC/TOS Guideline for the Management of Overweight and Obesity in Adults: A Report of the American College of Cardiology/American Heart Association Task Force on Practice Guidelines and The Obesity Society.** Circulation. 2013 Nov 12. [Epub ahead of print]
- **The use of triptans for pediatric migraines.** Paediatr Drugs. 2010 Dec 1 ;12(6):379-89. doi: 10.2165/11532860-000000000-00000.
- **Intestinal microbiota, diet and health.** Br J Nutr. 2014 Feb ;111(3):387-402. doi: 10.1017/S0007114513002560. Epub 2013 Aug 12 .
- **Obesity alters gut microbial ecology.** Proc Natl Acad Sci U S A. 2005 Aug 2 ;102(31):11070-5. Epub 2005 Jul 20 .

- **The gut microbiota and its relationship to diet and obesity**
  Gut Microbes. May 1, 2012; 3(3)186
- **The mathematical relationship between dishware size and portion size.**
  Appetite. 2012 Feb ;58(1):299-302.doi10.1016/j.appet.2011.10.010. Epub 2011 Oct 25 .
- **Plate size and children's appetite: effects of larger dishware on self-served portions and intake.**
  Pediatrics. 2013 May ;131(5):e1451-8. doi: 10.1542/peds.2012-2330. Epub 2013 Apr 8 .
- **Use of portion-controlled entrees enhances weight loss in women.**
  Obes Res. 2004 Mar ;12(3):538-46.
- **Position of the American Dietetic Association: weight management.** J Am Diet Assoc. 2009 Feb ;109(2):330-46.
- **Portion control plate for weight loss in obese patients with type 2 diabetes mellitus: a controlled clinical trial.** Arch Intern Med. 2007 Jun 25 ;167(12):1277-83.
- **Dietetics majors' weight-reduction beliefs, behaviors, and information sources.**
  J Am Coll Health. 2001 Jan ;49(4):175-81.
- **Overweight and obesity - use of portion control in management.**
  Aust Fam Physician. 2010 Jun ;39(6):407-11.
- **A community intervention on portion control aimed at weight loss in low-income Mexican American women.**
  J Midwifery Womens Health. 2010 Jan-Feb ;55(1):60-4. doi: 10.1016/j.jmwh.2009.03.014.
- **What impact does plate size have on portion control?**
  J Am Diet Assoc. 2011 Sep ;111(9):1438. doi: 10.1016/j.jada.2011.07.027.
- **A portion-control plate was effective for weight loss in obese patients with type 2 diabetes mellitus.**
  ACP J Club. 2007 Nov-Dec ;147(3):68.
- **Efficacy of meal replacements versus a standard food-based diet for weight loss in type 2 diabetes: a controlled clinical trial.**
  Diabetes Educ. 2008 Jan-Feb ;34(1):118-27. doi: 10.1177/0145721707312463.
- **A randomized comparison of a commercially available portion-controlled weight-loss intervention with a diabetes self-management education program**
  Nutrition & Diabetes. Mar 2013; 3(3)e63
- **A randomized comparison of a commercially available portion-controlled weight-loss intervention with a diabetes self-management education program.**
  Nutr Diabetes. 2013 Mar 18 ;3:e63. doi: 10.1038/nutd.2013.3.
- **The SHED-IT weight loss maintenance trial protocol: a randomised controlled trial of a weight loss maintenance program for overweight and obese men.**
  Contemp Clin Trials. 2014 Jan ;37(1):84-97. doi: 10.1016/j.cct.2013.11.004. Epub 2013 Nov 15 .

- **Obesity in the United States – Dysbiosis from Exposure to Low-Dose Antibiotics?**
  Frontiers in Public Health. 2013; 1()
- **Flos Lonicera Ameliorates Obesity and Associated Endotoxemia in Rats through Modulation of Gut Permeability and Intestinal Microbiota**
  PLoS ONE. 2014; 9(1)
- **Obesity in the United States - dysbiosis from exposure to low-dose antibiotics?**
  Front Public Health. 2013 Dec 19 ;1:69. doi: 10.3389/fpubh.2013.00069. eCollection 2013.
- **[The role of gut microbiota in the pathogenesis of obesity].**
  Postepy Hig Med Dosw (Online). 2014 Jan 24 ;68(0):84-90. doi: 10.5604/17322693.1086419.
- **'The way to a man's heart is through his gut microbiota' - dietary pro- and prebiotics for the management of cardiovascular risk.**
  Proc Nutr Soc. 2014 Feb 4:1-14. [Epub ahead of print]
- **Geographical variation of human gut microbial composition.**
  Biol Lett. 2014 Feb 12 ;10(2):20131037. doi: 10.1098/rsbl.2013.1037. Print 2014
- **Flos Lonicera Ameliorates Obesity and Associated Endotoxemia in Rats through Modulation of Gut Permeability and Intestinal Microbiota.**
  PLoS One. 2014 Jan 24 ;9(1):e86117. doi: 10.1371/journal.pone.0086117. eCollection 2014.
- **Gastrointestinal hormones and the dialogue between gut and brain.**
  J Physiol. 2014 Mar 17. [Epub ahead of print]
- **Increasing trends in incidence of overweight and obesity over 5 decades.**
  Am J Med. 2007 Mar ;120(3):242-50.
- **Obesity in the United States - dysbiosis from exposure to low-dose antibiotics?**
  Front Public Health. 2013 Dec 19 ;1:69. doi: 10.3389/fpubh.2013.00069. eCollection 2013.
- **[The role of gut microbiota in the pathogenesis of obesity].**
  Postepy Hig Med Dosw (Online). 2014 Jan 24 ;68(0):84-90. doi: 10.5604/17322693.1086419.
- **'The way to a man's heart is through his gut microbiota' - dietary pro- and prebiotics for the management of cardiovascular risk.**
  Proc Nutr Soc. 2014 Feb 4:1-14. [Epub ahead of print]
- **Geographical variation of human gut microbial composition.**
  Biol Lett. 2014 Feb 12 ;10(2):20131037. doi: 10.1098/rsbl.2013.1037. Print 2014
- **Flos Lonicera Ameliorates Obesity and Associated Endotoxemia in Rats through Modulation of Gut Permeability and Intestinal Microbiota.**
  PLoS One. 2014 Jan 24 ;9(1):e86117. doi: 10.1371/journal.pone.0086117. eCollection 2014.
- **Gastrointestinal hormones and the dialogue between gut and brain.**

J Physiol. 2014 Mar 17. [Epub ahead of print]

- **Increasing trends in incidence of overweight and obesity over 5 decades.**
  Am J Med. 2007 Mar ;120(3):242-50.

- **Obesity in the United States - dysbiosis from exposure to low-dose antibiotics?**
  Front Public Health. 2013 Dec 19 ;1:69. doi: 10.3389/fpubh.2013.00069. eCollection 2013.

- **[The role of gut microbiota in the pathogenesis of obesity].**
  Postepy Hig Med Dosw (Online). 2014 Jan 24 ;68(0):84-90. doi: 10.5604/17322693.1086419.

- **'The way to a man's heart is through his gut microbiota' - dietary pro- and prebiotics for the management of cardiovascular risk.**
  Proc Nutr Soc. 2014 Feb 4:1-14. [Epub ahead of print]

- **Geographical variation of human gut microbial composition.**
  Biol Lett. 2014 Feb 12 ;10(2):20131037. doi: 10.1098/rsbl.2013.1037. Print 2014.

- **Flos Lonicera Ameliorates Obesity and Associated Endotoxemia in Rats through Modulation of Gut Permeability and Intestinal Microbiota.**
  PLoS One. 2014 Jan 24 ;9(1):e86117. doi: 10.1371/journal.pone.0086117. eCollection 2014.

- **Gastrointestinal hormones and the dialogue between gut and brain.**
  J Physiol. 2014 Mar 17. [Epub ahead of print]

- **Increasing trends in incidence of overweight and obesity over 5 decades.**
  Am J Med. 2007 Mar ;120(3):242-50.

- **Gut microbiota signatures predict host and microbiota responses to dietary interventions in obese individuals.**
  PLoS One. 2014 Mar 6 ;9(3):e90702. doi: 10.1371/journal.pone.0090702. eCollection 2014.

- **Diet Effects in Gut Microbiome and Obesity.**
  J Food Sci. 2014 Mar 12. doi: 10.1111/1750-3841.12397. [Epub ahead of print]

- **Mechanisms of changes in glucose metabolism and bodyweight after bariatric surgery.**
  Lancet Diabetes Endocrinol. 2014 Feb;2(2):152-164. doi: 10.1016/S2213-8587(13)70218-3. Epub 2014 Feb 3.

- **Partial substitution of carbohydrate intake with protein intake from lean red meat lowers blood pressure in hypertensive persons.**
  Am J Clin Nutr. 2006 Apr ;83(4):780-7.

- **Roux-en-Y gastric bypass in mice--surgical technique and characterisation.**
  Obes Surg. 2012 Jul ;22(7):1117-25. doi: 10.1007/s11695-012-0661-9.

- **Probing the mechanisms of the metabolic effects of weight loss surgery in humans using a novel mouse model system.**
  J Surg Res. 2013 Jan ;179(1):e91-8. doi: 10.1016/j.jss.2012.02.036. Epub 2012 Mar 10 .

- Food reward in the obese and after weight loss induced by calorie restriction and bariatric surgery.
  Ann N Y Acad Sci. 2012 Aug ;1264:36-48. doi: 10.1111/j.1749-6632.2012.06573.x. Epub 2012 May 22 .
- The importance of the gut microbiota after bariatric surgery.
  Nat Rev Gastroenterol Hepatol. 2012 Oct ;9(10):590-8. doi: 10.1038/nrgastro.2012.161. Epub 2012 Aug 28 .
- Weight-independent effects of roux-en-Y gastric bypass on glucose homeostasis via melanocortin-4 receptors in mice and humans.
  Gastroenterology. 2013 Mar ;144(3):580-590.e7. doi: 10.1053/j.gastro.2012.11.022. Epub 2012 Nov 15 .
- Development and Verification of a Mouse Model for Roux-en-Y Gastric Bypass Surgery with a Small Gastric Pouch
  PLoS ONE. 2013; 8(1)
- Development and verification of a mouse model...
- Development and verification of a mouse model for Roux-en-Y gastric bypass surgery with a small gastric pouch.
  PLoS One. 2013 ;8(1):e52922. doi: 10.1371/journal.pone.0052922. Epub 2013 Jan 11 .
- Hyperglycemia and what to do about it.
  EMS World. 2013 Sep ;42(9):68-77.
- Metabolic consequences of chronic sleep restriction in rats: changes in body weight regulation and energy expenditure.
  Physiol Behav. 2012 Oct 10 ;107(3):322-8. doi: 10.1016/j.physbeh.2012.09.005. Epub 2012 Sep 17 .
- Piromelatine, a novel melatonin receptor agonist, stabilizes metabolic profiles and ameliorates insulin resistance in chronic sleep restricted rats.
  Eur J Pharmacol. 2014 Jan 30;727C:60-65. doi: 10.1016/j.ejphar.2014.01.037. [Epub ahead of print]
- Reproductive function of the male obese Zucker rats: alteration in sperm production and sperm DNA damage.
  Reprod Sci. 2014 Feb ;21(2):221-9. doi: 10.1177/1933719113493511. Epub 2013 Jun 25 .
- Visceral adiposity influences glucose and glycogen metabolism in control and hyperlipidic-fed animals.
  Nutr Hosp. 2013 Mar-Apr ;28(2):545-52. doi: 10.3305/nh.2013.28.2.6181.
- Green tea catechins prevent obesity through modulation of peroxisome proliferator-activated receptors.
  Sci China Life Sci. 2013 Sep ;56(9):804-10. doi: 10.1007/s11427-013-4512-2. Epub 2013 Jul 12 .
- Periodontal innate immune mechanisms relevant to obesity.
  Mol Oral Microbiol. 2013 Oct ;28(5):331-41. doi: 10.1111/omi.12035. Epub 2013 Aug 5 .
- Neuroimaging of gastric distension and gastric bypass surgery.
  Appetite. 2013 Dec ;71:459-65. doi: 10.1016/j.appet.2013.07.002. Epub 2013 Aug 9 .
- The snacking rat as model of human obesity: effects of a free-choice high-fat high-sugar diet on meal patterns.

Int J Obes (Lond). 2013 Aug 27. doi: 10.1038/ijo.2013.159. [Epub ahead of print]

- **Oxidized lipids activate autophagy in a JNK-dependent manner by stimulating the endoplasmic reticulum stress response.**
Redox Biol. 2013 Jan 26 ;1(1):56-64. doi: 10.1016/j.redox.2012.10.003. eCollection 2013.

- **The effects of dietary saturated fat on basal hypothalamic neuroinflammation in rats.**
Brain Behav Immun. 2014 Feb ;36:35-45. doi: 10.1016/j.bbi.2013.09.011. Epub 2013 Sep 25 .

- **Stress and eating behaviors.**
Minerva Endocrinol. 2013 Sep ;38(3):255-67.

- **Obesity accelerates ovarian follicle development and follicle loss in rats.**
Metabolism. 2014 Jan ;63(1):94-103. doi: 10.1016/j.metabol.2013.09.001. Epub 2013 Oct 14 .

- **Effect of insulin-resistance on circulating and adipose tissue MMP-2 and MMP-9 activity in rats fed a sucrose-rich diet.**
Nutr Metab Cardiovasc Dis. 2014 Jan 10. pii: S0939-4753(13)00198-1. doi: 10.1016/j.numecd.2013.08.007. [Epub ahead of print]

- **Assessment of Androgen Replacement Therapy for Erectile Function in Rats with Type 2 Diabetes Mellitus by Examining Nitric Oxide-Related and Inflammatory Factors.**
J Sex Med. 2014 Jan 28. doi: 10.1111/jsm.12447. [Epub ahead of print]

- **Effect of fructooligosaccharides fraction from Psacalium decompositum on inflammation and dyslipidemia in rats with fructose-induced obesity.**
Nutrients. 2014 Jan 29 ;6(2):591-604. doi: 10.3390/nu6020591.

- **Spexin is a novel human peptide that reduces adipocyte uptake of long chain fatty acids and causes weight loss in rodents with diet-induced obesity.**
Obesity (Silver Spring). 2014 Feb 18. doi: 10.1002/oby.20725. [Epub ahead of print]

- **Obesity as malnutrition: the role of capitalism in the obesity global epidemic.**
Am J Hum Biol. 2012 May-Jun ;24(3):261-76. doi: 10.1002/ajhb.22253. Epub 2012 Mar 2 .

- **Delayed diagnosis of abdominal mass due to morbid obesity.**
Acta Clin Belg. 2011 Mar-Apr ;66(2):137-8.

- **Conserved Shifts in the Gut Microbiota Due to Gastric Bypass Reduce Host Weight and Adiposity**
NIHPA Author Manuscripts. Mar 27, 2013; 5(178)178ra41

- **Conserved shifts in the gut microbiota due to gastric bypass reduce host weight and adiposity.**
Sci Transl Med. 2013 Mar 27 ;5(178):178ra41. doi: 10.1126/scitranslmed.3005687.

- **Bariatric surgery relieves type 2 diabetes and modulates inflammatory factors and coronary endothelium eNOS/iNOS expression in db/db mice.**

Can J Physiol Pharmacol. 2014 Jan ;92(1):70-7. doi: 10.1139/cjpp-2013-0034. Epub 2013 Oct 21 .

- **Vitamin D status before Roux-en-Y and efficacy of prophylactic and therapeutic doses of vitamin D in patients after Roux-en-Y gastric bypass surgery.**
  Obes Surg. 2009 May ;19(5):590-4. doi: 10.1007/s11695-008-9698-1. Epub 2008 Oct 11 .
- **Decreased Physical Activity Attributable to Higher Body Mass Index Influences Fibromyalgia Symptoms.**
  PM R. 2014 Feb 15. pii: S1934-1482(14)00075-6. doi: 10.1016/j.pmrj.2014.02.007. [Epub ahead of print]
- **Prevalence and risk factors for gallstone disease.**
  Surg Laparosc Endosc Percutan Tech. 2004 Oct ;14(5):250-3.
- **Gallstones, gallbladder disease, and pancreatitis: cross-sectional and 2-year data from the Swedish Obese Subjects (SOS) and SOS reference studies.**
  Am J Gastroenterol. 2003 May ;98(5):1032-41.
- **Osteoarthrosis**
  Canadian Family Physician. Jul 1984; 30()1503
- **Sleep restriction in adolescents: forging the path towards obesity and diabetes?**
  Sleep. 2013 Jun 1 ;36(6):813-4. doi: 10.5665/sleep.2694.
- **Obstructive sleep apnea is a predictor of abnormal glucose metabolism in chronically sleep deprived obese adults.**
  PLoS One. 2013 May 29 ;8(5):e65400. doi: 10.1371/journal.pone.0065400. Print 2013 .
- **Ghrelin and its interactions with growth hormone, leptin and orexins: implications for the sleep-wake cycle and metabolism.**
  Sleep Med Rev. 2014 Feb ;18(1):89-97. doi: 10.1016/j.smrv.2013.04.003. Epub 2013 Jun 29 .
- **Nocturnal ghrelin, ACTH, GH and cortisol secretion after sleep deprivation in humans.**
  Psychoneuroendocrinology. 2006 Sep ;31(8):915-23. Epub 2006 Jun 30 .
- **Metabolic and endocrine effects of sleep deprivation.**
  Essent Psychopharmacol. 2005 ;6(6):341-7.
- **The impact of sleep deprivation on food desire in the human brain.**
  Nat Commun. 2013 ;4:2259. doi: 10.1038/ncomms3259.
- **Stress and eating behaviors.**
  Minerva Endocrinol. 2013 Sep ;38(3):255-67.
- **Sleep deprivation and obesity in shift workers in southern Brazil.**
  Public Health Nutr. 2013 Oct 29:1-5. [Epub ahead of print]
- **Changes in children's sleep duration on food intake, weight, and leptin.**
  Pediatrics. 2013 Dec ;132(6):e1473-80. doi: 10.1542/peds.2013-1274. Epub 2013 Nov 4 .
- **[Night work and health of nurses and midviwes--a review].**
  Med Pr. 2013 ;64(3):397-418.

- **Piromelatine, a novel melatonin receptor agonist, stabilizes metabolic profiles and ameliorates insulin resistance in chronic sleep restricted rats.**
  Eur J Pharmacol. 2014 Jan 30;727C:60-65. doi: 10.1016/j.ejphar.2014.01.037. [Epub ahead of print]
- **The prevention and treatment of overweight and obesity. Summary of the advisory report by the Health Council of The Netherlands.**
  Neth J Med. 2004 Jan ;62(1):10-7.
- **Stress and the inflammatory process: a major cause of pancreatic cell death in type 2 diabetes**
  Diabetes, Metabolic Syndrome and Obesity: Targets and Therapy. 2014; 7()25
- **Non-Alcoholic Fatty Liver Disease (NAFLD) in Obesity**
  Journal of Clinical and Diagnostic Research : JCDR. Jan 2014; 8(1)62
- **Assessing the relationship between obesity and asthma in adolescent patients: a review**
  Adolescent Health, Medicine and Therapeutics. 2013; 4()39
- **Stress and the inflammatory process: a major cause of pancreatic cell death in type 2 diabetes.**
  Diabetes Metab Syndr Obes. 2014 Feb 3;7:25-34. eCollection 2014.
- **Role of the Microbiome in Energy Regulation and Metabolism.**
  Gastroenterology. 2014 Feb 18. pii: S0016-5085(14)00219-4. doi: 10.1053/j.gastro.2014.02.008. [Epub ahead of print]
- **Healthy weight regulation and eating disorder prevention in high school students: a universal and targeted web-based intervention.**
  J Med Internet Res. 2014 Feb 27 ;16(2):e57. doi: 10.2196/jmir.2995.
- **Non-Alcoholic Fatty Liver Disease (NAFLD) in Obesity.**
  J Clin Diagn Res. 2014 Jan ;8(1):62-6. doi: 10.7860/JCDR/2014/6691.3953. Epub 2013 Jan 12 .
- **Assessing the relationship between obesity and asthma in adolescent patients: a review.**
  Adolesc Health Med Ther. 2013 Feb 18;4:39-49. eCollection 2013.
- **Outcome of pulmonary embolism and clinico-radiological predictors of mortality: Experience from a university hospital in Saudi Arabia**
  Annals of Thoracic Medicine. Jan-Mar 2014; 9(1)18
- **The genetic and metabolic determinants of cardiovascular complications in type 2 diabetes: recent insights from animal models and clinical investigations.**
  Can J Diabetes. 2013 Oct ;37(5):351-8. doi: 10.1016/j.jcjd.2013.08.262.
- **Differences and similarities in development of corneal nerve damage and peripheral neuropathy and in diet-induced obesity and type 2 diabetic rats.**
  Invest Ophthalmol Vis Sci. 2014 Mar 3 ;55(3):1222-30. doi: 10.1167/iovs.13-13794.
- **Outcome of pulmonary embolism and clinico-radiological predictors of mortality: Experience from a university hospital in Saudi Arabia.**

Ann Thorac Med. 2014 Jan ;9(1):18-22. doi: 10.4103/1817-1737.124420.

- **Insulin-like growth factor-II: its role in metabolic and endocrine disease.**
  Clin Endocrinol (Oxf). 2014 Mar 5. doi: 10.1111/cen.12446. [Epub ahead of print]
- **Evolution of GLP1 and GLP1 receptor.**
  J Mol Endocrinol. 2014 Mar 5. [Epub ahead of print]
- **The Number of Metabolic Abnormalities Associated with the Risk of Gallstones in a Non-diabetic Population**
  PLoS ONE. 2014; 9(3)
- **The Number of Metabolic Abnormalities Associated with the Risk of Gallstones in a Non-diabetic Population.**
  PLoS One. 2014 Mar 5 ;9(3):e90310. doi: 10.1371/journal.pone.0090310. eCollection 2014.
- **Gastrointestinal morbidity in obesity.**
  Ann N Y Acad Sci. 2014 Mar 6. doi: 10.1111/nyas.12385. [Epub ahead of print]
- **Beyond the Role of Dietary Protein and Amino Acids in the Prevention of Diet-Induced Obesity**
  International Journal of Molecular Sciences. Jan 2014; 15(1)1374
- **Beyond the role of dietary protein and amino acids in the prevention of diet-induced obesity.**
  Int J Mol Sci. 2014 Jan 20 ;15(1):1374-91. doi: 10.3390/ijms15011374.
- **Weight loss interventions for chronic asthma.**
  Cochrane Database Syst Rev. 2012 Jul 11 ;7:CD009339. doi: 10.1002/14651858.CD009339.pub2.
- **Long-term effects of low-fat diets either low or high in protein on cardiovascular and metabolic risk factors: a systematic review and meta-analysis**
  Nutrition Journal. 2013; 12()48
- **Effect of a 6-month vegan low-carbohydrate ('Eco-Atkins') diet on cardiovascular risk factors and body weight in hyperlipidaemic adults: a randomised controlled trial**
  BMJ Open. 2014; 4(2)
- **Long term weight maintenance after advice to consume low carbohydrate, higher protein diets - A systematic review and meta analysis.**
  Nutr Metab Cardiovasc Dis. 2013 Dec 20. pii: S0939-4753(13)00301-3. doi: 10.1016/j.numecd.2013.11.006. [Epub ahead of print]
- **WITHDRAWN: Advice on low-fat diets for obesity.**
  Cochrane Database Syst Rev. 2008 Jul 16 ;(3):CD003640. doi: 10.1002/14651858.CD003640.pub2.
- **Long-term effects of low-fat diets either low or high in protein on cardiovascular and metabolic risk factors: a systematic review and meta-analysis.**
  Nutr J. 2013 Apr 15 ;12:48. doi: 10.1186/1475-2891-12-48.
- **Effect of an energy-restricted, high-protein, low-fat diet relative to a conventional high-carbohydrate, low-fat diet on weight loss,**

body composition, nutritional status, and markers of cardiovascular health in obese women.
Am J Clin Nutr. 2005 Jun ;81(6):1298-306.

- **Effect of a 6-month vegan low-carbohydrate ('Eco-Atkins') diet on cardiovascular risk factors and body weight in hyperlipidaemic adults: a randomised controlled trial.**
  BMJ Open. 2014 Feb 5 ;4(2):e003505. doi: 10.1136/bmjopen-2013-003505.
- **Glucose uptake by the brain on chronic high-protein weight-loss diets with either moderate or low amounts of carbohydrate.**
  Br J Nutr. 2014 Feb ;111(4):586-97. doi: 10.1017/S0007114513002900.
- **Diet-induced weight loss: the effect of dietary protein on bone.**
  J Acad Nutr Diet. 2014 Jan ;114(1):72-85. doi: 10.1016/j.jand.2013.08.021. Epub 2013 Oct 30 .
- **Human chorionic gonadotropin (HCG) treatment of obesity.**
  Arch Intern Med. 1977 Feb ;137(2):151-5.
- **Human Chorionic Gonadotropin (HCG) in the Treatment of Obesity**
  The Western Journal of Medicine. Dec 1977; 127(6)461
- **Toxicity of Weight Loss Agents**
  Journal of Medical Toxicology. Jun 2012; 8(2)145
- **HCG: Yet another fraudulence**
  Journal of Pharmacy & Bioallied Sciences. Jul-Sep 2012; 4(3)255
- **Where can I find information on the use of human chorionic gonadotrophin (HCG) for weight loss?**
  J Am Diet Assoc. 2010 Dec ;110(12):1960. doi: 10.1016/j.jada.2010.10.032.
- **Human chorionic gonadotropin (HCG) in the treatment of obesity: a critical assessment of the Simeons method.**
  West J Med. 1977 Dec ;127(6):461-3.
- **Toxicity of weight loss agents.**
  J Med Toxicol. 2012 Jun ;8(2):145-52. doi: 10.1007/s13181-012-0213-7.
- **HCG: Yet another fraudulence.**
  J Pharm Bioallied Sci. 2012 Jul ;4(3):255-6. doi: 10.4103/0975-7406.99068.
- **Ineffectiveness of human chorionic gonadotropin in weight reduction: a double-blind study.**
  Am J Clin Nutr. 1976 Sep ;29(9):940-8.
- **Human chorionic gonadotrophin and weight loss. A double-blind, placebo-controlled trial.**
  S Afr Med J. 1990 Feb 17 ;77(4):185-9.
- **Effect of the human chorionic gonadotropin diet on patient outcomes.**
  Ann Pharmacother. 2013 May ;47(5):e23. doi: 10.1345/aph.1R755. Epub 2013 Apr 19 .
- **Immunohistochemical and ultrastructural changes in rat fat tissue related to the local hCG injection.**
  Eur Rev Med Pharmacol Sci. 2013 Nov ;17(22):3103-10.

- The prevention and treatment of overweight and obesity. Summary of the advisory report by the Health Council of The Netherlands.
  Neth J Med. 2004 Jan ;62(1):10-7.
- By the way, doctor. I've had pain and burning near the entrance to my vagina for a long time. My doctor says it's probably vulvodynia. What can you tell me about this condition? How is it treated?
  Harv Womens Health Watch. 2010 Feb ;17(6):8.
- By the way, doctor. I've seen a lot of Internet ads for Hoodia, a natural supplement that suppresses your appetite. What do you know about it? Does it work, is it safe?
  Harv Womens Health Watch. 2008 Aug ;15(12):8.
- By the way, doctor. I've been trying to lose weight for a long time and nothing seems to work. What do you know about the HCG diet?
  Harv Womens Health Watch. 2010 May ;17(9):8.
- Where can I find information on the use of human chorionic gonadotrophin (HCG) for weight loss?
  J Am Diet Assoc. 2010 Dec ;110(12):1960. doi: 10.1016/j.jada.2010.10.032.
- Stress and the inflammatory process: a major cause of pancreatic cell death in type 2 diabetes.
  Diabetes Metab Syndr Obes. 2014 Feb 3;7:25-34. eCollection 2014.
- Role of the Microbiome in Energy Regulation and Metabolism.
  Gastroenterology. 2014 Feb 18. pii: S0016-5085(14)00219-4. doi: 10.1053/j.gastro.2014.02.008. [Epub ahead of print]
- Healthy weight regulation and eating disorder prevention in high school students: a universal and targeted web-based intervention.
  J Med Internet Res. 2014 Feb 27 ;16(2):e57. doi: 10.2196/jmir.2995.
- Non-Alcoholic Fatty Liver Disease (NAFLD) in Obesity.
  J Clin Diagn Res. 2014 Jan ;8(1):62-6. doi: 10.7860/JCDR/2014/6691.3953. Epub 2013 Jan 12 .
- Assessing the relationship between obesity and asthma in adolescent patients: a review.
  Adolesc Health Med Ther. 2013 Feb 18;4:39-49. eCollection 2013.
- The genetic and metabolic determinants of cardiovascular complications in type 2 diabetes: recent insights from animal models and clinical investigations.
  Can J Diabetes. 2013 Oct ;37(5):351-8. doi: 10.1016/j.jcjd.2013.08.262.
- Differences and similarities in development of corneal nerve damage and peripheral neuropathy and in diet-induced obesity and type 2 diabetic rats.
  Invest Ophthalmol Vis Sci. 2014 Mar 3 ;55(3):1222-30. doi: 10.1167/iovs.13-13794.
- Outcome of pulmonary embolism and clinico-radiological predictors of mortality: Experience from a university hospital in Saudi Arabia.

Ann Thorac Med. 2014 Jan ;9(1):18-22. doi: 10.4103/1817-1737.124420.

- **Insulin-like growth factor-II: its role in metabolic and endocrine disease.**
Clin Endocrinol (Oxf). 2014 Mar 5. doi: 10.1111/cen.12446. [Epub ahead of print]
- **Evolution of GLP1 and GLP1 receptor.**
J Mol Endocrinol. 2014 Mar 5. [Epub ahead of print]
- **The Number of Metabolic Abnormalities Associated with the Risk of Gallstones in a Non-diabetic Population.**
PLoS One. 2014 Mar 5 ;9(3):e90310. doi: 10.1371/journal.pone.0090310. eCollection 2014.
- **Gastrointestinal morbidity in obesity.**
Ann N Y Acad Sci. 2014 Mar 6. doi: 10.1111/nyas.12385. [Epub ahead of print]
- **Beyond the role of dietary protein and amino acids in the prevention of diet-induced obesity.**
Int J Mol Sci. 2014 Jan 20 ;15(1):1374-91. doi: 10.3390/ijms15011374.
- **Weight loss interventions for chronic asthma.**
Cochrane Database Syst Rev. 2012 Jul 11 ;7:CD009339. doi: 10.1002/14651858.CD009339.pub2.
- **WITHDRAWN: Advice on low-fat diets for obesity.**
Cochrane Database Syst Rev. 2008 Jul 16 ;(3):CD003640. doi: 10.1002/14651858.CD003640.pub2.
- **Long term weight maintenance after advice to consume low carbohydrate, higher protein diets - A systematic review and meta analysis.**
Nutr Metab Cardiovasc Dis. 2013 Dec 20. pii: S0939-4753(13)00301-3. doi: 10.1016/j.numecd.2013.11.006. [Epub ahead of print]
- **Long-term effects of low-fat diets either low or high in protein on cardiovascular and metabolic risk factors: a systematic review and meta-analysis.**
Nutr J. 2013 Apr 15 ;12:48. doi: 10.1186/1475-2891-12-48.
- **Effect of an energy-restricted, high-protein, low-fat diet relative to a conventional high-carbohydrate, low-fat diet on weight loss, body composition, nutritional status, and markers of cardiovascular health in obese women.**
Am J Clin Nutr. 2005 Jun ;81(6):1298-306.
- **Effect of a 6-month vegan low-carbohydrate ('Eco-Atkins') diet on cardiovascular risk factors and body weight in hyperlipidaemic adults: a randomised controlled trial.**
BMJ Open. 2014 Feb 5 ;4(2):e003505. doi: 10.1136/bmjopen-2013-003505.
- **Glucose uptake by the brain on chronic high-protein weight-loss diets with either moderate or low amounts of carbohydrate.**
Br J Nutr. 2014 Feb ;111(4):586-97. doi: 10.1017/S0007114513002900.
- **Diet-induced weight loss: the effect of dietary protein on bone.**

J Acad Nutr Diet. 2014 Jan ;114(1):72-85. doi: 10.1016/j.
jand.2013.08.021. Epub 2013 Oct 30 .

- **Human chorionic gonadotropin (HCG) treatment of obesity.**
  Arch Intern Med. 1977 Feb ;137(2):151-5.
- **Human Chorionic Gonadotropin (HCG) in the Treatment
  of Obesity**
  The Western Journal of Medicine. Dec 1977; 127(6)461
- **Human chorionic gonadotropin (HCG) in the treatment of obesity:
  a critical assessment of the Simeons method.**
  West J Med. 1977 Dec ;127(6):461-3.
- **Where can I find information on the use of human chorionic
  gonadotrophin (HCG) for weight loss?**
  J Am Diet Assoc. 2010 Dec ;110(12):1960. doi: 10.1016/j.
  jada.2010.10.032.
- **Toxicity of weight loss agents.**
  J Med Toxicol. 2012 Jun ;8(2):145-52. doi: 10.1007/s13181-
  012-0213-7.
- **HCG: Yet another fraudulence**
  Journal of Pharmacy & Bioallied Sciences. Jul-Sep 2012; 4(3)255
- **HCG: Yet another fraudulence.**
  J Pharm Bioallied Sci. 2012 Jul ;4(3):255-6. doi: 10.4103/0975-
  7406.99068.
- **Ineffectiveness of human chorionic gonadotropin in weight
  reduction: a double-blind study.**
  Am J Clin Nutr. 1976 Sep ;29(9):940-8.
- **Human chorionic gonadotrophin and weight loss. A double-blind,
  placebo-controlled trial.**
  S Afr Med J. 1990 Feb 17 ;77(4):185-9.
- **Effect of the human chorionic gonadotropin diet on
  patient outcomes.**
  Ann Pharmacother. 2013 May ;47(5):e23. doi: 10.1345/aph.1R755.
  Epub 2013 Apr 19 .
- **Immunohistochemical and ultrastructural changes in rat fat
  tissue related to the local hCG injection.**
  Eur Rev Med Pharmacol Sci. 2013 Nov ;17(22):3103-10.
- **The prevention and treatment of overweight and obesity.
  Summary of the advisory report by the Health Council of The
  Netherlands.**
  Neth J Med. 2004 Jan ;62(1):10-7.
- **By the way, doctor. I've had pain and burning near the entrance
  to my vagina for a long time. My doctor says it's probably
  vulvodynia. What can you tell me about this condition? How is
  it treated?**
  Harv Womens Health Watch. 2010 Feb ;17(6):8.
- **By the way, doctor. I've seen a lot of Internet ads for Hoodia, a
  natural supplement that suppresses your appetite. What do you
  know about it? Does it work, is it safe?**
  Harv Womens Health Watch. 2008 Aug ;15(12):8.
- **By the way, doctor. I've been trying to lose weight for a long
  time and nothing seems to work. What do you know about
  the HCG diet?**

Harv Womens Health Watch. 2010 May ;17(9):8.

- **Where can I find information on the use of human chorionic gonadotrophin (HCG) for weight loss?**
  J Am Diet Assoc. 2010 Dec ;110(12):1960. doi: 10.1016/j. jada.2010.10.032.

- **High Prevalence of Normal Tests Assessing Hypercortisolism in Subjects with Mild and Episodic Cushing's Syndrome Suggests that the Paradigm for Diagnosis and Exclusion of Cushing's Syndrome Requires Multiple Testing**
  NIHPA Author Manuscripts. 2010 November; 42(12)874

- **Anti-obesity effects of gut microbiota are associated with lactic acid bacteria.**
  Appl Microbiol Biotechnol. 2013 Nov 14. [Epub ahead of print]

- **Probiotics improve outcomes after Roux-en-Y gastric bypass surgery: a prospective randomized trial.**
  J Gastrointest Surg. 2009 Jul ;13(7):1198-204. doi: 10.1007/s11605-009-0891-x. Epub 2009 Apr 18 .

- **Intestinal and gastric bypass. Changes in intestinal microecology after surgical treatment of morbid obesity in man.**
  Scand J Gastroenterol. 1981 ;16(5):681-7.

- **Anti-obesity effects of gut microbiota are associated with lactic acid bacteria.**
  Appl Microbiol Biotechnol. 2013 Nov 14. [Epub ahead of print]

- **Probiotics improve outcomes after Roux-en-Y gastric bypass surgery: a prospective randomized trial.**
  J Gastrointest Surg. 2009 Jul ;13(7):1198-204. doi: 10.1007/s11605-009-0891-x. Epub 2009 Apr 18.

- **Intestinal and gastric bypass. Changes in intestinal microecology after surgical treatment of morbid obesity in man.**
  Scand J Gastroenterol. 1981 ;16(5):681-7.

- **Glucose uptake by the brain on chronic high-protein weight-loss diets with either moderate or low amounts of carbohydrate.**
  Br J Nutr. 2014 Feb;111(4):586-97. doi: 10.1017/S0007114513002900.
  Lobley GE1, Johnstone AM1, Fyfe C1, Horgan GW2, Holtrop G2, Bremner DM1, Broom I3, Schweiger L4, Welch A4.

- **Obesity as malnutrition: the role of capitalism in the obesity global epidemic.**
  Am J Hum Biol. 2012 May-Jun;24(3):261-76. doi: 10.1002/ajhb.22253. Epub 2012 Mar 2 Wells JC. PMID: 22383142 [PubMed - indexed for MEDLINE]

- **Weight-reducing side effects of the antiepileptic agents topiramate and zonisamide.**
  Handb Exp Pharmacol. 2012;(209):433-66. doi: 10.1007/978-3-642-24716-3_20. Antel J1, Hebebrand J.PMID: 22249827

- **Drug-induced weight gain.**
  Drugs Today (Barc). 2005 Aug;41(8):547-55.
  Author information: Ness-Abramof R1, Apovian CM.
  PMID: 16234878 [PubMed - indexed for MEDLINE]

- **Alogliptin improves steroid-induced hyperglycemia in treatment-naïve Japanese patients with chronic kidney disease by decrease of plasma glucagon levels.**
  Med Sci Monit. 2014 Apr 10;20:587-93. doi: 10.12659/MSM.889872.
  Ohashi N1, Tsuji N1, Naito Y1, Iwakura T1, Isobe S1, Ono M1, Fujikura T1, Tsuji T1, Sakao Y2, Yasuda H1, Kato A2, Fujigaki Y1.
  PMID: 24717767 [PubMed - in process] PMCID: PMC3989946
- **Gut–Brain Axis: Regulation of Glucose Metabolism**
  Department of Endocrinology and Metabolic Diseases, Leiden University Medical Center, Leiden, The Netherlands.
  TNO-Quality of Life, Gaubius Laboratory, Leiden, the Netherlands.
  Department of Cardiology, Leiden University Medical Center, Leiden, the Netherlands
- **Gut peptides in the control of food intake**
  TH Moran
  Department of Psychiatry and Behavioral Sciences, Johns Hopkins University School of Medicine, Baltimore, MD, USA
- **Gut Hormones and Appetite Control**
  A. M. WREN and S. R. BLOOM
  Department of Metabolic Medicine, Imperial College London, London, England
- **Gastrointestinal satiety signals**
  OB Chaudhri, BCT Field and SR Bloom
  Department of Investigative Science, Imperial College London, Hammersmith Hospital, London, UK
- **Voices from within: gut microbes and the CNS**
  Paul Forsythe•Wolfgang A. Kunze
- **Mind-altering microorganisms: the impact of the gut microbiota on brain and behavior** John F. Cryan & Timothy G. Dinan
- **Microbes and the gut-brain axis**
  P. BERCIK, S. M. COLLINS & E. F. VERDU
  Farcombe Family Digestive Health Research Institute, McMaster University, Hamilton, Canada
- **Obesity and its associated disease: A role for microbiota?**
  Ali Bonakdar Tehrani, Behtash Ghazi Nezami 1,2, Andrew Gewirtz 3, and Shanthi Srinivasan1,2 1 Division of Digestive Diseases, Emory University,
  Center for Inflammation, Immunity & Infection and Department of Biology, Georgia State University, Atlanta GA USA
- **Brain Gut Microbiome Interactions and Functional Bowel**
- **Disorders**
  Emeran A. Mayer, Tor Savidge and Robert J. Shulman
  Oppenheimer Center for Neurobiology of Stress, Division of Digestive Diseases, David Geffen, School of Medicine at UCLA, Los Angeles, CA
  Department of Pathology & Immunology, Baylor College of Medicine, Houston, TX
  Texas Children's Microbiome Center, Department of Pathology, Texas Children's Hospital, Houston, TX, USA
  Department of Pediatrics, Baylor College of Medicine, Children's Nutrition Research Center, Texas Children's Hospital, Houston, TX

- **Short-Chain Fatty Acids Stimulate Glucagon-Like**
- **Peptide-1 Secretion via the G-Protein**
  Gwen Tolhurst, Helen Heffron, Yu Shan Lam, Helen E. Parker, Abdella M. Habib, Eleftheria Diakogiannaki, Jennifer Cameron, Johannes Grosse, Frank Reimann,
  And Fiona M. Gribble

BOOK REFERENCE:

- **Scientific Evidence for Musculoskeletal, Bariatric, and Sports Nutrition**
  Edited by Ingrid Kohlstadt
- **Handbook of Obesity, Clinical Application, Edited by George A Bray and Claude Bouchard, Second Edition**
- **Handbook of Obesity, Etiology and Pathophysiology, Edited by George A Bray and Claude Bouchard, Second Edition**
- **Lippincott's Illustrated Reviews Biochemistry, 3rd Edition**
- **Evaluation and Management of Obesity, Daniel H Bessesen, MD and Robert Kushner, MD**

JOURNAL REFERENCE:

Series of Obesity research journal by Obesity Society.

Follow us on twitter :

> https://twitter.com/SlimPlate

Like us on facebook :

> https://www.facebook.com/SlimPlate

Read weight loss blog by Dr Nwe at :

> www.aceweightloss.com

Register Dr. Nwe's Online Weight Loss Program at :

> http://www.slimplatesystem.com/register

www.ingramcontent.com/pod-product-compliance
Lightning Source LLC
Chambersburg PA
CBHW060959280326
41935CB00009B/763